Treating Arthritis Diet Book

The late MARGARET HILLS SRN trained as a nurse at St Stephen's Hospital in London, until her training was cut short by crippling heart disease and arthritis. Against all the odds she fought back, and went on to marry, have eight children and continue a long career as an industrial nurse. Her radical new treatment for arthritis is shared through The Margaret Hills Clinic, 1 Oaks Precinct, Caesar Road, Kenilworth, Warwickshire CV8 1DP (tel. 01926 854 783). She wrote several bestselling books based on her experience: *Treating Arthritis: The drug-free way*, *Treating Arthritis: More ways to a drug-free life*, *Treating Arthritis Exercise Book* (with Janet Horwood) and *Cider Vinegar*, all published by Sheldon Press.

D0809848

Overcoming Common Problems Series

Selected titles

A full list of titles is available from Sheldon Press,
36 Causton Street, London SW1P 4ST and on our website at
www.sheldonpress.co.uk

The Assertiveness Handbook
Mary Hartley

Assertiveness: Step by step
Dr Windy Dryden and Daniel Constantinou

Backache: What you need to know
Dr David Delvin

Body Language: What you need to know
David Cohen

Calm Down
Paul Hauck

The Cancer Survivor's Handbook
Dr Terry Priestman

The Candida Diet Book
Karen Brody

Cataract: What you need to know
Mark Watts

The Chronic Fatigue Healing Diet
Christine Craggs-Hinton

The Chronic Pain Diet Book
Neville Shone

Cider Vinegar
Margaret Hills

The Complete Carer's Guide
Bridget McCall

The Confidence Book
Gordon Lamont

Confidence Works
Gladeana McMahon

Coping Successfully with Pain
Neville Shone

Coping Successfully with Panic Attacks
Shirley Trickett

Coping Successfully with Period Problems
Mary-Claire Mason

Coping Successfully with Psoriasis
Christine Craggs-Hinton

Coping Successfully with Ulcerative Colitis
Peter Cartwright

Coping Successfully with Varicose Veins
Christine Craggs-Hinton

Coping Successfully with Your Hiatus Hernia
Dr Tom Smith

Coping Successfully with Your Irritable Bowel
Rosemary Nicol

Coping with Age-related Memory Loss
Dr Tom Smith

Coping with Birth Trauma and Postnatal Depression
Lucy Jolin

Coping with Bowel Cancer
Dr Tom Smith

Coping with Candida
Shirley Trickett

Coping with Chemotherapy
Dr Terry Priestman

Coping with Childhood Allergies
Jill Eckersley

Coping with Childhood Asthma
Jill Eckersley

Coping with Chronic Fatigue
Trudie Chalder

Coping with Coeliac Disease
Karen Brody

Coping with Compulsive Eating
Ruth Searle

Coping with Diabetes in Childhood and Adolescence
Dr Philippa Kaye

Coping with Diverticulitis
Peter Cartwright

Coping with Down's Syndrome
Fiona Marshall

Coping with Dyspraxia
Jill Eckersley

Coping with Eating Disorders and Body Image
Christine Craggs-Hinton

Coping with Epilepsy in Children and Young People
Susan Elliot-Wright

Coping with Family Stress
Dr Peter Cheevers

Overcoming Common Problems Series

Coping with Gout
Christine Craggs-Hinton

Coping with Hay Fever
Christine Craggs-Hinton

Coping with Hearing Loss
Christine Craggs-Hinton

Coping with Heartburn and Reflux
Dr Tom Smith

Coping with Kidney Disease
Dr Tom Smith

Coping with Life after Stroke
Dr Mareeni Raymond

Coping with Macular Degeneration
Dr Patricia Gilbert

Coping with a Mid-life Crisis
Derek Milne

Coping with Polycystic Ovary Syndrome
Christine Craggs-Hinton

Coping with Postnatal Depression
Sandra L. Wheatley

Coping with Radiotherapy
Dr Terry Priestman

Coping with Snoring and Sleep Apnoea
Jill Eckersley

Coping with a Stressed Nervous System
Dr Kenneth Hambly and Alice Muir

Coping with Strokes
Dr Tom Smith

Coping with Suicide
Maggie Helen

Coping with Tinnitus
Christine Craggs-Hinton

Coping with Your Partner's Death: Your
bereavement guide
Geoff Billings

The Depression Diet Book
Theresa Cheung

Depression: Healing emotional distress
Linda Hurcombe

Depressive Illness
Dr Tim Cantopher

Eating for a Healthy Heart
Robert Povey, Jacqui Morrell and Rachel Povey

Every Woman's Guide to Digestive Health
Jill Eckersley

The Fertility Handbook
Dr Philippa Kaye

The Fibromyalgia Healing Diet
Christine Craggs-Hinton

Free Your Life from Fear
Jenny Hare

Free Yourself from Depression
Colin and Margaret Sutherland

A Guide to Anger Management
Mary Hartley

Heal the Hurt: How to forgive and move on
Dr Ann Macaskill

Help Your Child Get Fit Not Fat
Jan Hurst and Sue Hubberstey

Helping Children Cope with Anxiety
Jill Eckersley

Helping Children Cope with Change and Loss
Rosemary Wells

Helping Children Cope with Grief
Rosemary Wells

How to Approach Death
Julia Tugendhat

How to Be a Healthy Weight
Philippa Pigache

How to Beat Pain
Christine Craggs-Hinton

How to Cope with Difficult People
Alan Houel and Christian Godefroy

How to Get the Best from Your Doctor
Dr Tom Smith

How to Make Life Happen
Gladeana McMahon

How to Stop Worrying
Dr Frank Tallis

How to Talk to Your Child
Penny Oates

The IBS Healing Plan
Theresa Cheung

Is HRT Right for You?
Dr Anne MacGregor

Letting Go of Anxiety and Depression
Dr Windy Dryden

Living with Angina
Dr Tom Smith

Living with Asperger Syndrome
Dr Joan Gomez

Living with Autism
Fiona Marshall

Living with Bipolar Disorder
Dr Neel Burton

Living with Birthmarks and Blemishes
Gordon Lamont

Overcoming Common Problems Series

Living with Crohn's Disease
Dr Joan Gomez

Living with Eczema
Jill Eckersley

Living with Fibromyalgia
Christine Craggs-Hinton

Living with Food Intolerance
Alex Gazzola

Living with Gluten Intolerance
Jane Feinmann

Living with Grief
Dr Tony Lake

Living with Loss and Grief
Julia Tugendhat

Living with Osteoarthritis
Dr Patricia Gilbert

Living with Osteoporosis
Dr Joan Gomez

Living with Rheumatoid Arthritis
Philippa Pigache

Living with Schizophrenia
Dr Neel Burton and Dr Phil Davison

Living with a Seriously Ill Child
Dr Jan Aldridge

Living with Sjögren's Syndrome
Sue Dyson

Losing a Baby
Sarah Ewing

Losing a Child
Linda Hurcombe

The Multiple Sclerosis Diet Book
Tessa Buckley

Osteoporosis: Prevent and treat
Dr Tom Smith

Overcoming Agoraphobia
Melissa Murphy

Overcoming Anorexia
Professor J. Hubert Lacey, Christine Craggs-Hinton
and Kate Robinson

Overcoming Anxiety
Dr Windy Dryden

Overcoming Back Pain
Dr Tom Smith

Overcoming Depression
Dr Windy Dryden and Sarah Opie

Overcoming Emotional Abuse
Susan Elliot-Wright

Overcoming Hurt
Dr Windy Dryden

Overcoming Insomnia
Susan Elliot-Wright

Overcoming Jealousy
Dr Windy Dryden

**Overcoming Panic and Related Anxiety
Disorders**
Margaret Hawkins

Overcoming Procrastination
Dr Windy Dryden

Overcoming Shyness and Social Anxiety
Ruth Searle

Overcoming Tiredness and Exhaustion
Fiona Marshall

Overcoming Your Fear of Flying
Professor Robert Bor, Dr Carina Eriksen and
Margaret Oakes

Reducing Your Risk of Cancer
Dr Terry Priestman

Safe Dieting for Teens
Linda Ojeda

The Self-Esteem Journal
Alison Waines

Simplify Your Life
Naomi Saunders

Stammering: Advice for all ages
Renée Byrne and Louise Wright

Stress-related Illness
Dr Tim Cantopher

Ten Steps to Positive Living
Dr Windy Dryden

Think Your Way to Happiness
Dr Windy Dryden and Jack Gordon

The Thinking Person's Guide to Happiness
Ruth Searle

**Tranquillizers and Antidepressants: When to
start them, how to stop**
Professor Malcolm Lader

The Traveller's Good Health Guide
Dr Ted Lankester

Treating Arthritis Diet Book
Margaret Hills

Treating Arthritis: The drug-free way
Margaret Hills and Christine Horner

Treating Arthritis: More ways to a drug-free life
Margaret Hills

Understanding Obsessions and Compulsions
Dr Frank Tallis

When Someone You Love Has Depression
Barbara Baker

Overcoming Common Problems

Treating Arthritis Diet Book

MARGARET HILLS, SRN

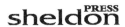

First published in Great Britain in 1986 as *Curing Arthritis Cookbook*

Sheldon Press
36 Causton Street
London SW1P 4ST

British Library Cataloguing-in-Publication Data
A catalogue record for this book
is available from the British Library

ISBN 978–0–85969–997–6

3 5 7 9 10 8 6 4

Typeset by Fakenham Photosetting Ltd
First printed and bound in Great Britain by
Clays Ltd, St Ives plc
Reprinted and bound in Great Britain by
Ashford Colour Press

*For my husband, Ivan, and our children,
Michael, Christine, Graham, Sally, Clive,
Peter, Bill and Mary.*

Contents

Acknowledgements   xi

Foreword   xiii

 1 The Value of Food and its Sources   1

 2 An Acid-Free Diet for the Arthritic   5

 3 Breakfast Dishes   15

 4 Hors-d'oeuvres   19

 5 Soups   23

 6 Fish Dishes   29

 7 Savouries and Sandwiches   41

 8 Salads   47

 9 Meatless Dishes   53

10 Meat Dishes   59

11 Poultry and Game   65

12 Sweets and Desserts   69

13 Cakes and Biscuits   75

Acknowledgements

My special thanks go to my daughter, Christine, for helping in the preparation and typing of this book.

Foreword

This book is a companion to my previous book entitled *Treating Arthritis – the Drug-Free Way*. In that, I told how I suffered the excruciating pain of arthritis for sixteen years – locked in every joint with both osteo- and rheumatoid arthritis – and how, having tried numerous so-called cures and diets, I eventually devised a diet and treatment for myself that rid me of all signs of arthritis in twelve months. That book also explained how I now give talks throughout the Midlands telling people what diet and treatment can be adopted for the relief of cure of arthritis, and the wonderful successes I have seen as the result of these talks and in the running of a busy clinic in Coventry.

Requests have come in day after day asking for a book containing 'acid-free' recipes and in response to these requests, I have decided to create this book of simple menus, bearing in mind that the majority of arthritics are elderly, many live alone, and although they like variety in their food, do not want to be bothered with elaborate recipes and preparation methods. I hope they will enjoy the following menus as much as I have enjoyed compiling them.

Margaret Hills, SRN

1

The Value of Food and its Sources

The human body can be likened to a plant which, if given the correct food, will thrive and produce beautiful leaves and flowers but, if not, will wither and die. It is of great benefit to know how different foods act on our bodies and where we can find these foods.

To keep healthy, the body needs an adequate intake of seven different elements – proteins, fats, carbohydrates, vitamins and minerals, water, fibre, and trace elements.

Protein

This is the material the body uses for growth and repair. Every cell in the body contains protein and if an adequate amount is not taken in each day the body cells break down, bringing about a state of 'dis-ease' in the individual. Protein also helps to regulate body metabolism. This means that it helps us to get the best possible value from the food we eat. It assists in the process of absorption. Protein is found mainly in the following foods – eggs, milk, cheese, cereals, pulses, nuts, meat.

Fats

There are two kinds of fat, namely animal and vegetable. Animal fats are found in meat and all dairy products and vegetable fats are found in vegetable margarines and oils. Fats help to supply heat and energy in the body and some also supply fat-soluble vitamins.

Carbohydrates

These are starchy foods that are flesh formers, and are mainly found in bread and potatoes, cereals and their products.

Vitamins and Minerals

These exist in small quantities in most animal and vegetable foods. The detrimental effects of a diet lacking in vitamins is very evident in the elderly and sometimes, too, in the young. Refined flours and cereals are sadly lacking in vitamins and minerals, as are white rice, cornflour, sago, tapioca, meat extracts, bacon, tinned and preserved meats, lard and margarine made from vegetable oils. Vitamins are found abundantly in egg yolk, cod liver oil and animal fats generally, and in the outer layers of cereals, which are removed by certain processes of milling. The 100 per cent wholemeal flour is best for our use, as is brown unpolished rice.

Cooking green vegetables with soda destroys the vitamins utterly. They should be cooked in as little water as possible and the water either drunk afterwards or used to make gravy in order to save the precious water-soluble vitamins contained therein.

Water

Water, of course, is most essential to our well-being; without it we cannot live. It is a wonderful body cleanser and we should drink lots of it every day.

Fibre

Fibre has come to the fore recently as being of very great value in the absorption of food and the regulation of peristalsis (bowel movement).

Trace Elements

Trace elements are another vital ingredient of our diet although at this moment in time little is known about their actual function in the prevention of disease.

A good all-round diet of milk, cheese, eggs, fish, meat or poultry, 100 per cent wholemeal bread, brown rice, and lots of vegetables and fruit, will supply the body with all the above ingredients to remain in a state of health.

Meat

Many people think that this is the only really nourishing food. This is a great mistake. Eating too much meat can cause a lot of health problems, especially for those who do not lead an active life, and it should be used in moderation especially by those with a tendency to arthritis and rheumatism. In fact, I recommend that beef and pork be cut out altogether because these meats are full of old fibrous tissue which contains uric acid, and when this meat is ingested a state of acidosis is set up in the body. This makes things worse for the unfortunate arthritis or rheumatism sufferer, who has already got a body full of acid.

Vegetables

Far too few vegetables are used. A stew is the most economical dish there is; the long slow cooking of the cheapest cuts of meat brings out the flavour, and all the goodness from the vegetables that are cooked with the meat is retained. A stew is an excellent dish for the arthritic; it requires little attention and can be prepared in the morning and left to cook slowly all day. It is tasty, nourishing and economical.

Cheese

This is the most valuable of foods. It is a highly concentrated protein food and is better value than meat or fish and lower in price. For example, 450 g (1 lb) cheese is about equal to 900 g (2 lbs) meat. It takes 4.5 l (1 gallon) milk to make 450 g (1 lb) cheese, which is equal in body-building value to 900 g (2 lbs) steak.

Grated cheese is a useful addition to salads and other foods that have little nourishment, but because of the lactic acid it contains, arthritics are advised to substitute cottage cheese as much as possible. This cheese is highly recommended because the lactic acid has been removed and the protein, vitamins and minerals are highly concentrated.

Fruits

Fruits in particular contain those vital trace elements necessary to ward off disease. They should be eaten regularly and in abundance, but arthritics should exclude citrus fruits such as oranges, lemons, grapefruits and their juices, rhubarb, tomatoes and strawberries from the diet because of the citric acid content. However, plenty of apples, peaches, pears, bananas, apricots and melons may be eaten.

2

An Acid-Free Diet for the Arthritic

Foods to have and those to avoid

At last people are beginning to realize that 'you are what you eat'. There is an ever-increasing awareness and interest today in healthier eating habits, and not before time. The age of refined white flour and refined sugar is gradually coming to an end and people are beginning to appreciate the value of wholemeal bread and unrefined sugar products.

Bread

Bread, being the staff of life, is most important in the daily diet. Everybody needs it every day.

For many thousands of years, bread has been one of our staple foods. In medieval times, the poor ate brown bread – it was the cheapest – while their richer brothers ate white bread. To obtain white flour the wheat had to go through a process of milling and sieving to remove all the bran and husk and this was very expensive, which the poorer people could not afford. As these processes became mechanized, white bread became cheaper and soon everybody was eating this and the sales of brown and wholemeal bread plummeted until very little was produced at all. But now, as a result of better education and increased interest in the foods we eat, there is a slow but sure return to the consumption of wholemeal bread.

The types of bread available in our shops today are determined first and foremost by the flour used. All flour starts out brown; it contains protein and is high in dietary fibre. This is a very valuable ingredient in our diet. It is not digested by our bodies and passes straight through, but it helps to keep the digestive system healthy by supplying the roughage needed to encourage peristalsis (bowel movement).

The milling and refining necessary to obtain white flour removes certain parts of the wheat grain and in doing so removes some of the nutrients. White flour is fortified with the B vitamins, thiamin and niacin, and the minerals iron and calcium, but it is still lacking in dietary fibre and other natural elements, including protein. Thiamin and niacin are vital to the body – they help to convert the food we eat into energy. Iron forms a part of red blood cells and it also helps to transport oxygen round the body – it helps in the prevention of anaemia and its associated illnesses. Calcium is needed by the body for sound teeth and healthy gums. It helps in the formation of bones and prevents them becoming brittle. It is also needed by the skin, hair and eyes, to keep them healthy.

The amount of protein in white flour varies according to how much it has been milled and refined. A regular supply of protein is very necessary because it forms the structure of most of the cells in the body and these are constantly growing or being replaced. There are several varieties of white breads and all are made from fortified white flour. The standard white loaf is the most common. It is a tin loaf and is sold sliced or unsliced in different thicknesses. There are other varieties of white bread, such as Farmhouse, Crusty Bloomer, Danish Baguette and Baton. There is also the Hi-fibre white loaf which is made from fortified white flour to which vegetable protein has been added.

None of the foregoing white breads can equal the higher dietary value of *100 per cent wholemeal bread*. This is made from flour that contains all of the wheat grain. The flour is either made by the traditional method of crushing the grain between two large millstones or by the modern methods of milling. Wholemeal bread is much coarser and more crumbly than other brown breads because all the outer part of the grain is included in the flour. Wholemeal bread is not additionally fortified with vitamins and minerals, as these are present naturally. It is available as large or small loaves or rolls and the following are the different varieties available.

100 per cent rustic wholemeal bread

This is made from whole wheat grains that have been crushed into flakes, rather than milled into flour. The flakes are soaked for a short while to soften them before the dough is made and this makes a smoother, moister mixture. The shaped dough is rolled in crushed wheat flakes before proving and baking to give added texture and flavour. The bread itself rises better than ordinary wholemeal, has a good even texture and is not crumbly. The flavour is full and nutty. Rustic bread is an excellent source of dietary fibre – even higher than ordinary wholemeal bread. The variety of rustic wholemeal breads available includes loaves, cobs, baguettes and rolls.

Granary or malted mixed grain bread

This is a brown bread to which crushed wheat and rye grains have been added, together with malted whole wheat. This makes the bread coarser and more moist and improves its keeping quality. It is darker in colour and nuttier in flavour than other brown breads.

Wheatgerm breads

These are made from flour to which about 10 per cent of wheatgerm has been added. Wheatgerm is normally removed from flour during milling because it is high in fat and the fat has a tendency to go rancid during storage. Modern techniques now make it possible to remove the wheatgerm and treat it to prevent rancidity so that it can be added back to the flour. It is an important addition because it contains significant amounts of the B vitamins. Wheatgerm bread cuts well, and has a delicious wheaty flavour.

Pitta bread

This traditional Greek bread is made from a white or wholemeal dough that contains only a small amount of yeast. After a short fermentation, the dough is divided and each piece is rolled out, then baked in a special high temperature oven. When the bread is removed from the oven, it is full of steam and looks like a rugby ball, but this steam leaks out to leave the bread in its characteristic flat oval shape. Pitta bread is usually warmed in the oven or under the grill before serving with a paté or dip. It may also be cut in half and split to make a pocket which can be filled with roast or grilled meats and salads.

Storage

To retain the freshness of bread for as long as possible, wrap it loosely in a polythene bag and keep it in a cool, dry place. Loose wrapping is important as it allows a small amount of air to circulate around the loaf. A tight wrapping will trap moisture and encourage the development of mould. Bread should not be kept in the refrigerator because although this will prevent mould, it will tend to dry the bread out. If a loaf has gone a little stale you can freshen it up by brushing the top lightly with milk and baking it in the oven at 190°C/375°F/Gas Mark 5, for 10–15 minutes until it is crisp. Allow it to cool before slicing or the inside will squash. Alternatively, slice it thickly before warming, then wrap in foil and bake for 15 minutes.

Freezing

Almost all bread can be frozen successfully as long as it is packed properly. Wrap the bread well in foil or polythene, ensuring the wrapping is tight. Most breads will keep well for at least six weeks, with the exception of crusty loaves and rolls. Occasionally the crust lifts off when the bread is thawed. Sliced bread is an excellent standby to have in the freezer as it can be taken out a few slices at a time and either toasted from the frozen state or defrosted for sandwiches and snacks. To defrost bread, loosen the wrappers and leave a loaf at room temperature for about three hours. Allow 1½ hours for rolls.

Hints and tips

1 If you have to make packed lunches, make up a batch of sandwiches and place in the freezer. Take out and defrost individually as required. Add salad ingredients when thawed.
2 Use moist fillings in sandwiches so you do not need butter or margarine.
3 Never throw away stale bread. There are many uses that stale bread can be put to, so not one crumb needs to be wasted.
• Make breadcrumbs from it and store in the freezer in a plastic bag. Use for coatings, stuffings, crunchy toppings and delicious fruit puddings such as fruit charlottes.

- Try making good old-fashioned bread-and-margarine pudding or summer pudding to use up stale sliced bread.
- If you have a lot of crusts or stale bread, dry them out in a cool oven, then crush them finely and use as coatings for grilled or oven-baked food.
- Pep up soup with crunchy croutons: cut small cubes of stale bread and bake them in the oven until crisp and golden brown.
- A crisp casserole topping is delicious. Arrange squares of sliced bread spread with vegetable margarine – margarined side up – on top of casserole, the oven temperature should be 200°C/400°F/ Gas Mark 6. Try beating some mustard into the margarine before spreading.
- Use breadcrumbs to thicken soups: stir a spoonful at a time into hot home-made soup over a gentle heat until it achieves the required consistency.

Weekly dietary requirements

The following is a weekly guideline of food intake for an adult healthy person to maintain optimum health and vitality. It is an acid-free diet as far as possible and will help in the treatment of arthritis, rheumatism and associated diseases, and should go a long way towards preventing the occurrence of these diseases in the healthy person. It is also a low-fat diet which is invaluable in the treatment of any form of heart trouble, e.g. angina, high blood pressure, varicose veins, etc., and also in the treatment of gall bladder and cystitis conditions, when combined with a low salt intake.

Bread

One week's supply, though people performing manual labour may need more, is approximately 1.5kg (3 lbs) of wholewheat bread.

Meat

Approximately 750 g (1¾ lbs) after trimming. Eat lean meat only, but exclude beef and pork, and any of their derivatives – bacon, ham, pork paté, for example, also corned beef or any meat derived from beef. The following meats can be included in the weekly diet – lamb, chicken, veal, duck, turkey, lamb's liver, lamb's heart, rabbit – in fact, any young meats.

Fish

Approximately 275 g (10 oz) each week. White fish, cooked in any way except fried in batter, is excellent. If eating tinned fish, the oil should be first poured away.

Vegetables

Approximately 1.5kg (3 lbs) of fresh green vegetables each week and the best way to eat them is raw or very lightly cooked in a little boiling water. When vegetables are cooked for too long or in a lot of water, the water soluble vitamins are lost, so to prevent this they should be cooked in the minimum amount of water and the water afterwards drunk as a cocktail or used in the gravy. This procedure will retain those valuable vitamins. When possible I serve vegetables raw – a variety such as cauliflower, red peppers, green peppers, apples, celery, spring onion – all washed, dried, chopped finely and tossed in a French dressing (made with cider vinegar instead of malt vinegar). Brown rice and cashew nuts add protein and carbohydrates to this healthy concoction.

Potatoes

Approximately 1.5kg (3½ lbs) potatoes are permitted unless, of course, there is an obese condition, in which case the amount of potatoes is reduced until the desired weight is reached.

Eggs

Approximately three eggs weekly is adequate, because eggs contain a lot of cholesterol and when this builds up in the body it can lead to angina, varicose veins, and the more serious associated diseases, such as coronary heart disease and strokes. The number of eggs that go into cakes should also be counted and reckoned as part of the limit of three per person.

Fats and Oils

Polyunsaturated margarine should always be used and approximately 150g (5 oz) per week is an adequate amount. The weekly intake may also include 100g (4oz) low-fat cottage cheese and about 300ml (½ pint) unsaturated oil.

Fruit

Approximately 1.25kg (2½lbs) fresh fruit. Do not eat the citrus fruits, e.g. oranges, lemons, grapefruits, pineapples, rhubarb, strawberries, plums – these contain citric acid and when taken in conjunction with carbohydrates set up a condition of uric acid in the system, leading to rheumatism and arthritis amongst other diseases. The juices of these fruits should also be avoided.

Milk

Skimmed or dried milk is best and approximately 1.2l (2 pints) per week is adequate.

Dried pulses

Peas, beans, lentils provide second-class protein. The recommended amount is 40g (1½oz) per week.

Wholewheat rice

Approximately 450g (1lb) per week.

Cakes, biscuits, pastries

An amount of 200g (7oz) per week is acceptable unless the person is overweight and wants to reduce, in which case these should be cut out altogether.

Yoghurt

This is basically cured or fermented milk. It is an excellent source of vitamins, minerals and protein, but like milk it is a dairy product and unless the 'very low fat' variety is available it should be avoided. Live yoghurt contains bacterias that have not been killed by heat treatment. Ninety per cent of all yoghurt bought is live, whether sold in a supermarket or health food store.

Live yoghurt has the same nutritional value as dead yoghurt (which is heat-treated). Live yoghurt contains bacteria that can survive in the stomach and kill organisms that cause diarrhoea, according to the findings of the Food Research Institute in Reading under the direction of Professor Michael Gurr.

Natural yoghurt is a live yoghurt that contains no colourings, preservatives, stabilizers or non-milk thickeners and is not heat-treated. It can contain added fruit, vitamins or sugar. *'U.H.T.'*, *'Pasteurized'* or *'Sterilized'* yoghurts are not live and have been heat-treated for a longer shelf life.

Some popular yoghurts contain a very high quantity of sugar and of course these should not be consumed by people on a reducing diet, or by arthritics. The 'very low fat' yoghurts are acceptable occasionally for arthritis sufferers, but since dairy products are best avoided altogether, they should not be indulged in regularly.

How to make your own yoghurt
1 Sterilize all equipment in boiling water.
2 Heat 600 ml (1 pint) skimmed milk to 43°C (blood heat).
3 Blend in 1 tablespoon of natural unfruited yoghurt and pour into a warmed vacuum flask.
4 Seal and leave for seven hours.

Using 600 ml (1 pint) of skimmed milk makes approximately 580 g (1¼ lbs) of natural yoghurt which is acceptable to arthritic sufferers, unless they are overweight and have to watch their calories.

Cider vinegar

The health-giving properties in cider vinegar are numerous. It is made from the juice of organically grown apples and is an excellent source of potassium and minerals, namely chlorine, magnesium, calcium, sulphur, iron, fluorine, silicon, phosphorus and many trace elements. Patients with arthritis will find the following dosage most beneficial:

One teaspoon of clear honey dissolved in a tumbler of hot water to which 1 dessertspoon cider vinegar is added. Take three times daily.

Honey

Honey is an excellent energy giver and should be used instead of sugar wherever possible. It is full of naturally occurring vitamins and minerals and is excellent for calming the nerves and promoting sleep, amongst many other attributes.

Drinks

The only drinks I have found to be non-acid-forming are blended vegetable drinks, e.g. carrot, cabbage, etc.; also apple juice, sold in cartons from supermarkets and health food shops, and water. Water is an excellent blood cleaner and supplies many minerals to the body. Plenty should be drunk every day. All short drinks are acid – sherry, gin, whisky, martini, etc., as are all table wines and citrus fruit drinks, such as orange juice, lemon, grapefruit and lime juice. All these should be avoided.

Tea and coffee are both acid-forming. Tea should be taken weak, only one or two cups daily. Decaffeinated coffee may be taken freely, also herb teas.

Vegetable broths are excellent and can be taken hot or cold. A week's supply can be made and when cold can be frozen in small amounts and consumed when needed. Cabbage, cauliflower, parsnip, or any root or green vegetables are wonderful sources of potassium, iron and minerals.

3

Breakfast Dishes

In my opinion a pleasant, nourishing unhurried breakfast is a must – it sets the pace for the day's work. It is well worthwhile getting up half-an-hour earlier and giving oneself time to sit down, relax and enjoy a well-cooked breakfast before leaving for work. Getting to work ten minutes early will give you a leisurely start to the day and what a difference that will make!

Kedgeree

450 g (1 lb) cold cooked fish
50 g (2 oz) low-cholesterol
   margarine
1 teacup unpolished rice

2 eggs, hard-boiled
pepper and sea salt to taste
chopped parsley

Wash and boil the rice until tender, then strain, and put in a warm place to dry. Chop the eggs into irregular pieces. Remove all skin and bone from the fish and break it into small flakes. Melt the margarine in a saucepan and warm the fish, rice, and eggs in this for ten minutes. Season and pile on to a dish, garnishing with parsley.

Sardines on toast

4 slices of toast spread with
   low-cholesterol margarine
1 tin sardines
chopped parsley

15 g (½ oz) low cholesterol
   margarine
1 tablespoon skimmed milk
sea salt and pepper

Drain sardines of all oil. Melt the margarine in a pan, stir in the flaked sardines and warm through. Add the milk, heating through but not boiling. Serve on the toast, garnishing with parsley.

Kippers

kippers   pepper
low-cholesterol margarine

Trim off the heads and tails and plunge the kippers into boiling water. Drain and place on grill tray with a knob of margarine on each. Cook quickly under a hot grill, and just before serving add a shake of pepper.

Plain omelette

2 eggs, per person   sea salt and pepper
15 g (½ oz) low-cholesterol
    margarine

Break the eggs into a bowl, add salt and pepper to taste and beat lightly. Melt the margarine in an omelette pan or small frying pan. When sizzling, add the eggs and stir until they begin to thicken. Cook until a golden brown then tilt the pan and fold over about one-third of the omelette towards the centre. Fold over again, making a very loose roll and turn on to a warmed serving plate.

Stewed fresh fruit

225 g (8 oz) apples   150 ml (¼ pint) water
25–50 g (1–2 oz) honey

Peel and slice the apples. Measure the honey and water into a saucepan and stir over a low heat to dissolve the honey. Add the prepared fruit, cover with a lid and cook slowly until the fruit is tender. Draw the pan off the heat and allow to cool. Spoon fruit into a serving dish and chill until ready to serve.

Porridge

600 ml (1 pint) water   ¼ level teaspoon sea salt
2 rounded tablespoons medium
    oatmeal

The night before, measure the water, oatmeal and salt into a saucepan. Leave to soak overnight. *To cook,* bring to the boil stirring all the time. Lower the heat and leave to simmer for 15 minutes, stirring occasionally. Serve hot with skimmed milk and honey or a sprinkling of sea salt.

Mushroom on toast

100 g (4 oz) mushrooms
sea salt and pepper

25 g (1 oz) low-cholesterol margarine
2 slices wholemeal bread

Wash and trim the mushrooms, remove the stalks and place cap side down in a well-buttered baking dish. Season and dot with margarine. Cover, place in the centre of a hot oven (200°C/400°F/ Gas Mark 6) and bake for 15 minutes. Toast the bread. Lift the mushrooms on to the toast slices, pour on the juice from the baking dish and serve.

Muesli

1 tablespoon quick-cooking rolled oats
3 tablespoons water

1 large eating apple
1 tablespoon natural yoghurt
light muscovado sugar or honey

Soak oats in the water overnight. Wash and grate the apple and mix with the oats. Add yoghurt. A little sugar or honey may be added to taste.

NOTE: Muesli can be varied by adding chopped nuts or by varying the fruit. Try sultanas, raisins, apricots, pears, bananas, grapes, or peaches.

Muffins

75 g (3 oz) plain flour
175 g (6 oz) wholegrain flour
a pinch of sea salt
40 g (1½ oz) molasses

15 g (½ oz) baking powder
1 beaten egg
250 ml (8 fl oz) skimmed milk
15 g (½ oz) low-cholesterol margarine

Preheat oven to 200°C/400°F/Gas Mark 6. Sift together the flours and salt into a bowl. Stir in the molasses and baking powder. Beat in the egg, milk and margarine. Fill the well-greased tins of a tartlet tin with the batter. Bake in the oven for 20–25 minutes. Serve with margarine and honey or diabetic apricot jam.

Herrings with mustard sauce

4 fresh herrings
sea salt and pepper

300 ml (½ pint) mustard sauce
(see below)

Clean and scale the fish. Make three incisions on each side. Place on a greased grid under preheated grill and cook 3–4 minutes on each side. Season and serve with mustard sauce.

Mustard sauce

25 g (1 oz) low-cholesterol
   margarine
25 g (1 oz) wholemeal flour
300 ml (½ pint) skimmed milk
   or water

1 tablespoon made mustard
1 dessertspoon cider vinegar
sea salt and pepper

Melt margarine in saucepan, stir in the flour. Cook for a few minutes without browning. Add some of the liquid, stir and boil for a few minutes. Add salt and pepper, mustard and cider vinegar.

Bran and apricot compote

225 g (8 oz) bran
100 g (4 oz) canned
   apricots, drained

160 g (5½ oz) natural yoghurt
25 g (1 oz) light muscovado sugar

Divide the bran between four dishes. Dice the apricots and mix with the yoghurt and sugar. Pour over the bran and serve.
   NOTE: You can substitute other fruits such as peaches, pears, etc.

4

Hors d'oeuvres

This is a useful course. It helps to dull appetite and also it helps both to build a meal, or make a meal go further if you have unexpected guests. It is easy to get an hors d'oeuvre together quickly from the odd tins you have in your store-cupboard, and from eggs and the pickles and chutney in daily use. Choose any from the lists which follow, varying your garnish according to the season – watercress, mustard and cress, heart of lettuce leaves, freshly chopped chives, parsley, mint.

Shrimp cocktail

lettuce, a small quantity of
100 g (4 oz) shrimps
3 tablespoons olive oil

sea salt and pepper
1 tablespoon cider vinegar
paprika

Shred the lettuce and put a little into the bottom of small glasses. Arrange the shrimps on top. Put oil, salt, pepper and cider vinegar into a screw-topped jar and shake well until thoroughly blended. Pour over shrimps. Sprinkle with paprika and serve as cold as possible.

As variation, lobster, crab or prawns may be used in place of shrimps.

Crab or lobster canapés

Spread rounds of toasted wholemeal bread with finely chopped crab or lobster meat. Add sprinkle of sea salt, cayenne, paprika and moisten with a little home-made mayonnaise (see page 51) or thick white sauce made with skimmed milk (see page 38). Brown in a hot oven.

Cucumber with shrimps

1 cucumber
75 g (3 oz) pounded shrimps
paprika
25 g (1 oz) low-cholesterol
   margarine

1 dessertspoon yoghurt
cress
home-made mayonnaise (see
   page 51)

Cut the cucumber into 5-cm (2-inch) lengths. Peel these very carefully, and with a tube cutter cut out the seeds to form small cases. Pound the shrimps, paprika, margarine and seasoning together. Moisten with yoghurt. Pile into cases and serve cold, garnished with mayonnaise and cress.

Smoked salmon

Cut into tissue paper thin slices and accompany with brown bread spread with low-cholesterol margarine.

Tuna fish

Cut up the fish into thin slices. Arrange these in a little dish surrounded by finely minced parsley or chopped watercress, and place a little heap of chopped capers on top of each slice.

Kipper fillets

Sprinkle uncooked kipper fillets with cider vinegar, slice very thinly and serve with brown bread spread with low-cholesterol margarine. This is as delicious as smoked salmon.

Canapés of sardines

1 tin sardines
4 slices wholemeal bread
low-cholesterol margarine
home-made mayonnaise (see
   page 51)

chopped olive
watercress
beetroot, cubed

Drain sardines of oil. Toast the bread and spread with low-cholesterol margarine. Lay a sardine on each slice. Mash with mayonnaise and sprinkle with olive. Garnish with watercress and beetroot.

Cauliflower and eggs

cauliflower
parsley, finely minced

French dressing (see page 51)
3–4 eggs, hard-boiled

Cook the cauliflower and allow to cool. Carefully divide into small pieces. Arrange in the centre of a plate. Cover each piece with parsley and pour on the home-made French dressing. Slice the hard-boiled eggs and arrange around the cauliflower.

Celery

Cut the stalks of celery up into neat evenly-sized pieces. Fill them with one of the following:
  yoghurt, garnished with paprika
  mango chutney and cottage cheese
  finely minced chicken and cottage cheese

Mushroom canapés

Toast slices of wholemeal bread and cut into small rounds. Spread on one side with low-cholesterol margarine and add a few fried mushrooms. Season with sea salt and pepper and serve immediately.

Canapés of chicken

Allow per person:
1 round wholemeal bread
1 tablespoon minced cold
  chicken
low-cholesterol margarine for
  frying

1 teaspoon aspic jelly
sea salt and pepper to taste
home-made mayonnaise (see
  page 51)

Fry the rounds of bread in the margarine, drain and allow to cool. Heap the seasoned, minced chicken on top and put the aspic jelly in the centre. Pipe mayonnaise around and over the chicken.

Pear and cream cheese

2 ripe pears	1 teaspoon chopped onion
cider vinegar	sea salt and pepper
15 g (½ oz) walnuts, chopped	parsley
225 g (8 oz) cottage cheese	lettuce

Peel pears, halve them and remove cores. Brush with cider vinegar. Stir walnuts into cottage cheese, add onion and seasoning. Pile on to pear halves and arrange on a serving dish. Garnish with parsley and serve with lettuce and a well-flavoured French dressing (see page 51).

5

Soups

There is nothing like a good nourishing soup on a cold winter's day. All types of vegetables may be used. A hard-boiled egg chopped and added to the soup will provide good protein. Serve with wholemeal croutons for an excellent warming meal. A variety of garnishes may be added such as chopped chives, chopped parsley, sliced mushrooms, chopped watercress, green pepper, or very thin slices of cucumber.

Cauliflower and lettuce soup

750 g (1½ lbs) neck of lamb
3 young turnips
3 young carrots
3 small onions
1.2 l (2 pints) of water

1 small lettuce
½ cauliflower
450 g (1 lb) peas
parsley
a pinch of sea salt

Heat water in saucepan then add half the lamb. Add sea salt and bring to the boil. Skim carefully. Simmer for 1 hour and then add remainder of meat cut into small chops, also turnips and carrots diced, the onions cut small, and half the peas. Simmer for another ½ hour. Chop the lettuce and divide the cauliflower into sprigs. Chop the parsley. Add these ingredients to the soup with the rest of the peas and simmer for another ½ hour. Season and serve.

Macaroni soup

225 g (8 oz) each of turnip,
   carrots and onions
100 g (4 oz) macaroni
1 small beetroot

25 g (1 oz) parsley
50 g (2 oz) low-cholesterol
   margarine
1.2 l (2 pints) water
600 ml (1 pint) skimmed milk

23

Slice turnips, carrots and onions and bring them to the boil in the water. Break the macaroni small and cook in the milk according to the instructions on the packet. Cook beetroot in salted boiling water until soft. When the mixed vegetables are cooked, add the macaroni, parsley, beetroot (cut small) and margarine. Season to taste with sea salt and pepper, and serve hot.

Potato and leek soup

450 g (1 lb) potatoes, thinly sliced
4 leeks, sliced in 5-cm (2-inch) sections
1 stick celery, white part only

50 g (2 oz) low-cholesterol margarine
1 teaspoon sea salt
1.2 l (2 pints) stock or water

Melt margarine in saucepan. Stir potatoes, leeks and diced celery in this for 5 minutes, but do not brown. Sprinkle salt over vegetables and add stock. Simmer gently for 1½ hours. Serve with wholemeal toast cut into squares.

Lentil and rice soup

¾ teacup lentils
½ teacup wholegrain rice
1.75 l (3 pints) water
chicken stock cube

2 onions, finely chopped
1 carrot, grated
2 tablespoons minced parsley
sea salt to taste

Soak lentils for 24 hours, after washing them well. Add the stock cube to the water and bring to the boil, then add lentils, vegetables and rice. Simmer for 1½ hours. Season and serve.

Mulligatawny soup

1.2 l (2 pints) stock
2 onions
2 cooking apples
1 tablespoon wholemeal flour
sea salt to taste

25 g (1 oz) low-cholesterol margarine
1 teaspoon honey
½ teaspoon cider vinegar
few pieces of cold fowl, lean lamb or firm fish

Melt the margarine in a saucepan. Chop the onions and fry in the margarine until soft but not brown. Add the apples, chopped, and allow them to cook until very soft. Stir in the flour, then add the stock slowly and finally the honey. Simmer for 1 hour, then rub soup through a sieve. Put the soup back into the pan to heat. Cut the meat or fish into small pieces and add to the soup. Continue to cook for a few minutes until thoroughly heated through, but do not let the soup boil. Add the cider vinegar and serve, with boiled wholegrain rice as an accompaniment.

Scotch broth

900 g (2 lbs) neck of lamb
1.2 l (2 pints) water
1 onion
1 carrot, diced
1 turnip, diced

50 g (2 oz) pearl barley
bouquet garni
sea salt
1 teaspoon chopped parsley

Cut meat up finely, removing fat and skin, chop the bones and add to the water with onion, seasoning and bouquet garni. Allow to simmer gently for 1 hour. Strain and remove bones. Return to the saucepan with the barley, carrot and turnip. Simmer till carrot is tender. Put back some of the meat cut into neat pieces, season and add parsley just before serving.

Onion soup

3 Spanish onions
2 small onions
25 g (1 oz) low-cholesterol
   margarine
65 g (2½ oz) wholemeal flour

1.5 l (2½ pints) water
150 ml (¼ pint) skimmed milk
sea salt

Peel and slice the onions. Put into a saucepan with the margarine and cook for 5 minutes with the lid on. Add the water and salt. Boil until the onion is quite tender. Mix the flour smoothly with the milk, add to the soup and boil well. Season to taste and serve.

Carrot and turnip soup

2 carrots	1 oz low-cholesterol margarine
2 turnips	2 pints boiling water
1 leek	1 oz wholemeal flour
1 onion	½ pint skimmed milk
1 stick celery	½ teaspoonful honey
1 bay leaf	sea salt

Clean vegetables and cut into strips. Put them into a saucepan with the margarine and cook for 5 minutes with the lid on, shaking occasionally. Add the boiling water, bay leaf and honey, and boil gently until the carrot is tender. Mix the flour smoothly with the milk, stir into the soup, boil well and season.

Cabbage soup

1 good-sized cabbage	chopped parsley
4 carrots, sliced	2 cloves garlic
2 turnips, sliced	sea salt
1 leek, sliced	1.5 l (2½ pints) water
1 clove	

Shred the cabbage. Bring the water to the boil and add all the vegetables, the clove and 2 teaspoonfuls of sea salt. Simmer for 2 to 3 hours. About 30 minutes before serving, add parsley and garlic, chopped fine. Stir occasionally and serve accompanied by croutons of wholemeal toast.

Chicken soup

600 ml (1 pint) chicken stock	600 ml (1 pint) skimmed milk
50 g (2 oz) low-cholesterol margarine	1 tablespoon wholemeal flour
2 carrots, sliced	50–75 g (2–3 oz) soft wholemeal breadcrumbs
2 onions, sliced	sea salt to taste
2 sticks celery	

Cook the vegetables in the margarine for 2 to 3 minutes; add stock and breadcrumbs. Boil for 10 minutes and strain. Blend milk with 25 g (1 oz) low-cholesterol margarine and flour. Add to stock. Season with salt and serve hot.

Watercress soup

100 g (4 oz) watercress
1 tablespoon sunflower oil
600 ml (1 pint) chicken stock,
  or water with chicken stock
  cube added

15 g (½ oz) cornflour
150 ml (¼ pint) skimmed milk
sea salt and pepper

Wash the watercress. Reserve some small sprigs to garnish the soup, and chop the remaining leaves coarsely. Fry slowly for 2 to 3 minutes in the hot oil. Add the stock and bring to the boil, stirring. Simmer for about 15 minutes. Do not overcook. Rub through a sieve and return to the pan. Mix the cornflour smoothly with the milk and add to the purée. Cook for 3 minutes, stirring well until thick. Add seasoning. Garnish with sprigs of watercress.

Cauliflower soup

1 cauliflower
50 g (2 oz) low-cholesterol
  margarine
600 ml (1 pint) chicken
  stock
15 g (½ oz) cornflour

300 ml (½ pint) skimmed milk
sea salt and pepper
1 egg yolk

Wash the cauliflower and divide into sprigs. Toss these in half of the margarine without browning. Add stock and simmer gently until the cauliflower is cooked. Rub through a sieve and reheat. Blend cornflour and milk and stir into stock; cook for a further 5 minutes. Season. Just before serving add the beaten egg yolk and the remaining margarine.

6

Fish Dishes

Fish is very high in protein and contains essential vitamins and minerals. White fish in particular is very low in fat, therefore it should form part of any healthy varied diet. Current medical opinion recommends that we should reduce the total amount of fat we eat and have a higher proportion of polyunsaturated fat in the fat we do eat. As a higher proportion of the fat contained in white fish is polyunsaturated, it really does contribute to a healthier diet. White fish also contains vitamins A and D and the B group of vitamins, also calcium and iodine. Fish is a very versatile food which can be cooked in a variety of ways. Try to steer clear of frying, but if you do have to fry use polyunsaturated oils like sunflower or corn oil, and drain the fish thoroughly on kitchen paper before serving.

Poaching

This method of cooking fish can be done in fish stock or a court bouillon. Place the fish in a fish kettle or large saucepan and cover completely with stock or liquor. Add a dash of cider vinegar, some chopped parsley, a few slices of onion, peppercorns and a bay leaf. Bring the liquid to the boil and simmer gently, allowing approximately 8 minutes per 450 g (1 lb) weight of fish.

Grilling

Clean and prepare fish – thaw frozen fish; gut whole fresh fish and score each side of the body with three or four diagonal cuts. Brush the fish with a little melted polyunsaturated margarine. Allow 4–5 minutes for fillets and 5–6 minutes for whole fish, thick steaks and cutlets, then brush again with the melted margarine and cook for another 5–6 minutes. Fish is delicate, so only turn once.

Baking

Season fish with a little salt and pepper. Wrap loosely in foil with a little fish stock. Bake in a moderate oven 180°C/350°F/Gas Mark 4. Allow 25–30 minutes for whole fish and 10–20 minutes for steak or fillets. Whole fish can be stuffed if desired.

Braising

Wash, peel and finely chop a selection of vegetables, such as onions, celery, carrots, etc. Simmer for 4–5 minutes, drain and place in heat-proof dish. Lay fish on top and add a dash of cider vinegar and a little black pepper. Add fresh parsley and cover with fish stock. Cover dish and bake at 180°C/350°F/Gas Mark 4, for 25 minutes approximately.

Steaming

This is an excellent way of preparing whole fish fillets and thin cuts of fish. Place them on a plate or in a steamer over a pan of simmering water. Sprinkle with a little black pepper and brush with polyunsaturated margarine. Cook for 5–15 minutes depending on size.

Cooking fish in a microwave

Wrap thinner parts of fish in a piece of paper to prevent overcooking. Fish should be placed in a single layer in a cooking dish and covered with a lid or cling film. It should be cooked until it looks opaque and then left to stand in the covered dish for 5 minutes.

The following are some of the more popular fish available today.

White fish

Cod

This is a very popular fish. Its flesh is firm with a delicate flavour. Codling are sold whole and are delicious stuffed and baked. Cod fillets and cutlets can be poached, steamed, baked or grilled and served with a white or parsley sauce, made with skimmed milk and polyunsaturated margarine.

Carp

Steam or bake this rich-tasting fish. Stuff if desired.

Coley

Usually sold filleted and is cheaper than cod, but can be cooked as cod.

Haddock

This is delicious steamed or poached. Its flesh is firm and it has a stronger flavour than cod. It can be purchased smoked.

Hake

This can be treated just like cod or haddock and it is a very good fish to use in stews, soups and casseroles.

Halibut

This fish is mainly sold as steaks and is best cooked on the bone because of a tendency to dry out during cooking. Braising or poaching is recommended.

Plaice

Try this fish grilled or poached – it has a soft, mild-tasting flesh.

Skate

The wings of the skate are the only part of the fish eaten. They are delicious and unusual poached and baked, and served in a salad.

Whiting

Poaching and baking are most suitable for this fish. It is similar in appearance to cod and has a sweetly-flavoured flesh.

Dover sole/lemon sole

Both are flat fish. Dover sole is said to have the best flavour. Either is delicious grilled or poached.

Oily fish

Herring

This is a very popular fish with a rich-tasting flesh. Herrings can be bought whole or filleted and are delicious baked or grilled. They are cold-smoked to make kippers, and can also be lightly smoked to make bloaters.

Mackerel

Served with a cold salad, this is delicious grilled or baked.

Salmon

Wrap in foil before poaching or baking as it has a tendency to dry out. Serve hot or cold.

Trout

This is sold as whole fish and best grilled or baked.

Eel

There are two varieties – fresh water eel and the conger eel. The conger eel needs slow, gentle cooking because the flesh is hard and tough, but it is well flavoured and makes tasty stews and pies. The freshwater eel has firm, white, richly-flavoured flesh. The small ones can be used to make jellied eels. When smoked, they can be eaten cold as a starter, like smoked mackerel.

Sprat

The most common way of cooking is to fry, but the larger ones can be very tasty stuffed, rolled and baked.

Whitebait

Most commonly fried but can be grilled or baked.

Shellfish and other sea food

Prawns

These are sold cooked and ready peeled, both fresh and frozen. Delicious cold in salads or cocktails and hot in fish pies, sauces, etc.

Crabs

These are usually sold cooked, fresh or frozen. They contain two types of meat, well-flavoured brown meat and delicate white meat. The flesh can be used in cocktails, soups and omelettes, or served with sauces.

Lobsters

Lobsters are a luxury because they are fairly scarce. They are best served as simply as possible and can be eaten hot or cold, with a suitable sauce.

Cockles

These are usually sold cooked and shelled and are tasty in fish soups or pies. They can also be eaten plain or pickled – in cider vinegar.

Mussels

If mussels are bought alive, any shells that are not closed or which do not close when tapped should be discarded. If uncleaned, scrape off any barnacles and rinse in several changes of water before cooking. Cook in water or fish stock for 5 minutes. They can be served hot in soups, pies, or paella, or they can be served with cider vinegar.

Scallops

These are best poached or grilled and served hot with a sauce or cold with a salad.

Fish casserole

450 g (1 lb) flaked white fish, cooked in skimmed milk	450 g (1 lb) mashed potato
2 tablespoons plain yoghurt	1 beaten egg
sea salt and pepper	2 tablespoons skimmed milk
	25 g (1 oz) low-cholesterol margarine

Lightly oil a casserole dish. Mix fish with milk, yoghurt and seasoning and place in casserole. Mix potato with the egg and milk, season and place over the fish. Score the top with a fork. Cover and bake in oven 180°C/350°F/Gas Mark 4, for 20 minutes. Remove cover and dot with margarine. Grill until brown. Serve with cooked green beans or peas.

Poached cod

900 g (2 lbs) cod	cider vinegar
sea salt	parsley

Wash the fish well in salt and water, place it in hot water in a saucepan with a little cider vinegar and sea salt. Simmer very slowly until cooked, skimming occasionally. Allow 10 minutes per 450 g (1 lb) and 10 minutes over. Drain well, serve in a hot dish, garnish with parsley and serve with oyster or any other suitable sauce (see pages 38–40).

Cod with green sauce

1 medium-sized onion	1 tablespoon soft wholemeal breadcrumbs
2 tablespoons chopped parsley	
2 teaspoons capers	1 tablespoon cider vinegar
2–3 gherkins	sea salt and pepper
4 cod cutlets	1 tablespoon olive oil

Grate the onion and pound in a mortar together with the parsley, capers and chopped gherkins. Continue pounding until a smooth paste is achieved, add the breadcrumbs and continue to pound. Pour in the oil and mix well, then add the cider vinegar and season with pepper and salt if necessary. Put the fish into an ovenproof dish, season well and cover each piece of fish with the sauce. Cover the dish and bake for approximately 15 minutes just above centre of a moderately hot oven, 200°C/400°F/Gas Mark 6. Serve with boiled or jacket potatoes.

Stuffed whiting

6 medium-sized whiting
beaten egg

cocktail sticks

low-cholesterol margarine

For the stuffing
3 tablespoons wholemeal
   breadcrumbs
½ teaspoon mixed herbs

sea salt and pepper
1 teaspoon chopped onion

Trim the fish by opening and cleaning inside. Remove the eyes and wash the fish thoroughly. Make up stuffing of breadcrumbs, onion, herbs, and seasoning and bind with some of the egg. Stuff each fish and close the opening with thin skewers or cocktail sticks. Place in fireproof dish and brush the tops with beaten egg and sprinkle with crumbs. Dab with margarine and place under preheated grill until cooked through.

Stuffed and baked haddock

1 haddock
65 g (2½ oz) wholemeal
   breadcrumbs
1 dessertspoon chopped parsley
¼ teaspoon sea salt

1 dessertspoon chopped onion
50 g (2 oz) low-cholesterol
   margarine
1 egg
¼ teaspoon pepper

Clean and wipe the haddock; cut off the fins. Put the breadcrumbs into a bowl, rub the margarine into them and then add the parsley, onion, salt and pepper. Mix well. Beat the egg and bind the mixture with it. Press the stuffing into the haddock and close the end with a skewer. Place the fish in an oiled baking tin, dust on a little flour, and dot the top with pieces of margarine. Bake in a moderate oven. 180°C/350°F/Gas Mark 4, for 20 minutes. The haddock may be egged over and rolled in breadcrumbs before being baked. Serve with a white sauce (see page 38).

Stuffed and baked fillets of plaice

900 g (2 lbs) plaice fillets
15 g (½ oz) low-cholesterol
   margarine
15 g (½ oz) wholemeal flour
150 ml (¼ pt) skimmed milk

cider vinegar
sea salt and pepper
chopped parsley

For the veal stuffing
100 g (4 oz) wholemeal
   breadcrumbs
50 g (2 oz) low-cholesterol
   margarine
1 teaspoon chopped parsley

½ teaspoon mixed herbs
1 egg
sea salt and pepper

Make the veal stuffing: place into a bowl the breadcrumbs, margarine, chopped parsley and mixed herbs. Mix together with the beaten egg, season. Place a little stuffing on each fillet, roll up and place on a greased tin, sprinkling with a little cider vinegar. Bake slowly 170°C/325°F/Gas Mark 3, for approximately 15–20 minutes. Heat the margarine gently, remove from the heat and stir in the flour. Return to the heat and cook for a few minutes. Again, remove the pan from the heat and gradually blend in the cold milk. Bring to the boil and cook, stirring with a wooden spoon, until smooth. Season well. When cooked, place the fillets on a hot dish and coat them with the sauce. Garnish with chopped parsley.

Fish omelette

cold cooked fish
white sauce (see page 38)
3 eggs

25 g (1 oz) low-cholesterol
   margarine
skimmed milk
sea salt and cayenne pepper

Remove the skin and bone from the fish, flake it and add a little white sauce, seasoning well. Keep it hot. Beat the eggs thoroughly, melt the margarine in an omelette pan. When hot pour in the eggs, stir for a moment, then allow them to set. When cooked sufficiently, put the pan under the grill to brown on the top. Put in the fish, fold over and serve on a hot dish immediately.

Sole à la turque

1 sole
1 tablespoon wholemeal
   breadcrumbs
20 g (¾ oz) low-cholesterol
   polyunsaturated margarine
150 ml (¼ pint) peeled shrimps
1 egg, beaten

300 ml (½ pint) stock
1 shallot
½ teaspoon herbs
1 teaspoon chopped parsley
wholemeal breadcrumbs
sea salt and pepper

Skin the sole, remove head, tail and fins, wash thoroughly. Make an incision down the fish on one side and raise the fillets. Chop the shrimps and make a stuffing with the wholemeal breadcrumbs, 15 g (½ oz) margarine, chopped shallot, and herbs, moistened with the beaten egg. Place it in the fish, adding some small dabs of margarine. Place sole in an ovenproof dish and add stock. Bake at 180°C/350°F/Gas Mark 4 for 20 minutes. To serve, sprinkle on a few wholemeal crumbs and garnish with parsley.

Grilled herrings

4 herrings
corn oil

low-cholesterol margarine
mustard sauce (see page 39)

Remove the heads, wash herrings and clean thoroughly without breaking. Score the fish with a knife and brush with corn oil. Put under the grill and cook on both sides. Place on a hot dish with a small piece of margarine on each and serve with mustard sauce.

Poached mackerel

4 mackerel
sea salt

parsley sauce or fennel sauce
(see page 39)

Open the fish just enough to take out the roe, thoroughly cleanse the fish and the roe and replace it; remove the eyes. Place in salted water, just below boiling point, and simmer 8–10 minutes according to the size, taking care not to break the skin which will happen if cooked too fast. Place on a warm dish, garnish with parsley, and serve with parsley or fennel sauce.

Steamed trout with yoghurt

4 trout, gutted and cleaned
4 tablespoons cider vinegar

1 tablespoon fresh chopped
   parsley
1 teaspoon dried thyme

For the sauce
160 g (5½ oz) yoghurt
3 dessertspoons cider vinegar
½ teaspoon dried tarragon

1 teaspoon chives
2 tablespoons horseradish,
   grated

Place trout on large sheet of foil. Sprinkle with cider vinegar, parsley and thyme. Fold the foil up to form a parcel. Place parcel between two plates and stand them on a pan of boiling water. Steam until tender, approximately 10–15 minutes. Transfer to a hot serving dish. Put yoghurt, horseradish, cider vinegar, tarragon and chives into a small heatproof bowl, place the bowl over a pan of simmering water and stir until hot and creamy. Pour sauce over trout and serve immediately. This dish can also be served cold.

Baked salmon steaks

4 salmon steaks
chopped parsley
1 shallot, chopped

cider vinegar
sea salt and pepper
caper sauce (see page 40)

Place the steaks in an oiled baking dish, season with chopped parsley, shallot, sea salt, pepper and cider vinegar. Cover with oiled paper, and cook in a hot oven, 220°C/425°F/Gas Mark 7, for 10–15 minutes. Place on warm dish and serve with caper sauce.

White sauce

25 g (1 oz) wholemeal flour
25 g (1 oz) low-cholesterol
   margarine

300 ml (½ pint) skimmed milk
sea salt and pepper

Heat the margarine gently, remove from the heat and stir in the flour. Return to the heat and cook for a few minutes. Again, remove the pan from the heat and gradually blend in the cold milk. Bring to the boil and cook, stirring with a wooden spoon, until smooth. Season well.

NOTE: this is the foundation white sauce. By adding extra ingredients to this a great variety of sauces can be easily made.

Oyster sauce

300 ml (½ pint) white sauce
3 or 4 oysters
cider vinegar
sea salt
cayenne pepper
1 tablespoon yoghurt

Scald the oysters and remove the beards, add to the white sauce with their liquor. Season with salt, cayenne, and a little cider vinegar, and add the yoghurt. Serve with boiled fish and boiled poultry.

Mustard sauce

300 ml (½ pint) white sauce
1 dessertspoon made mustard
sea salt and pepper

Add the made mustard to the sauce and season. Serve with grilled herrings.

Parsley sauce

300 ml (½ pint) white sauce
sea salt and pepper
½ tablespoon chopped parsley

Chop and blanch the parsley, add to the sauce and season. Serve with boiled fish, rabbit, poultry, etc.

Fennel sauce

300 ml (½ pint) white sauce
½ tablespoon fennel
sea salt and pepper

Chop the fennel, add to the white sauce and season. Serve with boiled mackerel.

Caper sauce

300 ml (½ pint) white sauce
  using half skimmed milk
  and half stock)

sea salt and pepper
1 tablespoon capers

Add chopped capers to the white sauce and season. Serve with salmon.

7

Savouries and Sandwiches

Where pastry is mentioned make your own with wholemeal flour and low-cholesterol margarine. The crunchy, nutty texture is delicious and very good for you. Wholemeal flour contains all the goodness of the wheat; none of the husk is removed; it is very good for the digestion and also very beneficial for bowel movement.

SAVOURIES

Wholemeal shortcrust pastry

225 g (8 oz) wholemeal flour
  margarine
½ teaspoon sea salt

100 g (4 oz) low-cholesterol
cold water to mix

Sieve the flour and salt. Rub in the fat until the mixture resembles fine breadcrumbs, and mix with sufficient water to give a stiff dough. Roll out and use as required.

Sardines on toast

1 tin sardines
sea salt

toast spread with low-
  cholesterol margarine

Cut the toast in long pieces, same length as the sardines. Drain the sardines from the can and remove bones. Place one on each piece of toast and season with a little sea salt. Place under the grill for a few minutes and serve very hot.

Lamb and egg toast

2 eggs
2 tablespoons cooked lamb,
  minced

25 g (1 oz) low-cholesterol
  margarine
sea salt 4 rounds of toast
4 rounds of toast

Put the margarine, eggs, meat and seasoning into a saucepan and stir until the eggs become thick. Pile on the rounds of toast and serve hot.

Rice fritters

100 g (4 oz) brown rice
1 shallot
25 g (1 oz) low-cholesterol
  margarine
1 tablespoon sunflower oil

1 egg, beaten
chopped parsley
sea salt

Cook the rice in boiling salted water until cooked (about 30 minutes) and drain. Chop the shallot and fry lightly in margarine. Add the shallot to the rice with parsley, beaten egg and salt. Heat oil in a pan and fry the rice mixture in small cakes until golden brown. Serve with lettuce and a little French dressing (see page 51).

Stuffed mushrooms

225 g (½ lb) open mushrooms
lamb's liver, chopped
25–50 g (1–2 oz) wholemeal
  breadcrumbs
1 teaspoon chopped shallot,
  or spring onions, chopped

sea salt
skimmed milk
25 g (1 oz) low-cholesterol
  margarine
chopped parsley
croutons of wholemeal bread

Prepare the croutons by frying in sunflower oil and then keep them hot in the oven. Wash the mushrooms, peel, and remove the stalks. Chop up the liver. Mix together the liver, breadcrumbs, parsley, and onion; season with salt. Bind with a little skimmed milk. Fill the mushrooms with this mixture, put a piece of margarine on each, and bake for 15 minutes in an oiled baking dish at 180°C/350°F/Gas

Mark 4. Lift out carefully, place each mushroom on one of the fried croutons and serve very hot.

Potato and onion pie

900 g (2 lbs) potatoes
225 g (8 oz) onions

sea salt
50 g (2 oz) low-cholesterol
   margarine

Peel the potatoes thinly and slice 5 mm (¼-inch) thick. Peel and slice the onions. Cover with cold, salted water and bring to the boil. Simmer gently for about 5–7 minutes or until cooked. Drain well and dry. Layer the potatoes and onions in a greased shallow pie dish. Season each layer. Dot with margarine and brown under grill.

Potato and onion omelette

For each serving:
1 small onion, chopped
1 small potato
25 g (1 oz) low-cholesterol
   margarine

2 eggs, beaten
sea salt

Slice the potato and boil in salted water until cooked. Melt margarine in a frying pan and fry onion and diced cooked potato until browned. Season the eggs and pour over the onion and potato. Cook as for an ordinary omelette. Turn out on to a hot plate and serve.

Cottage cheese flan

20-cm (8-inch) cooked
   wholemeal pastry
   flan case
1 large onion
15 g (½ oz) low-cholesterol
   margarine
1 tablespoon capers

2 eggs
150 ml (¼ pint) skimmed milk
225 g (8 oz) cottage cheese
sea salt and pepper

Chop the onion finely and fry in margarine until golden brown. Add the chopped capers, beaten eggs, milk and cottage cheese.

Season. Pour into the flan case and bake in the oven, at 180°C/ 350°F/Gas Mark 4, for 20 minutes until set.

Walnut mince

50 g (2 oz) chopped walnuts
75 g (3 oz) wholemeal breadcrumbs
10 g (¼ oz) low-cholesterol margarine
a little sea salt

1 onion, chopped
1 teaspoon dried mixed herbs
150 ml (¼ pint) water or stock

Melt margarine in saucepan. Add nuts and chopped onion and stir until lightly browned. Add the breadcrumbs and seasonings together with water or stock. Simmer slowly for 15 minutes, then serve on wholemeal toast.

SANDWICHES

A good sandwich can constitute a good nourishing meal. Always use wholemeal bread and low-cholesterol margarine. A good protein filling such as chicken, cottage cheese, fish, eggs, nuts, is a must if the sandwich is a meal, rather than a snack. Combine this with lettuce, cucumber, celery, watercress, etc., and you have an excellent meal, so quick and easy to prepare.

Hints on preparing sandwiches

- Instead of slicing cold meat, mince the meat and then incorporate it with the low-cholesterol margarine, one-third margarine to two-thirds minced meat. This saves time and is more economical.
- Fish is best baked, or creamed with margarine.
- Add yoghurt as moistener for a fish or meat paste.
- Nuts should be minced or ground fine.
- Lettuce is a good accompaniment for most meats.

Savoury sandwiches

For a savoury sandwich, choose one of the following:

Cottage cheese and shredded lettuce

Cottage cheese and nuts, minced

Salmon and cucumber

Cottage cheese and watercress

Dates (chopped) and walnuts (ground)

Cottage cheese and chopped celery

Celery and cashew nuts (ground)

Celery and almonds (ground)

Flaked fish with grated celery, or plain yoghurt

Cucumber with mustard and cress

Cucumber with chopped watercress

Cucumber with chopped capers

Cucumber with chicken

Cucumber with home-made chutney (using cider vinegar instead of malt vinegar)

Sardines boned and mixed to a paste with low-cholesterol margarine, seasoned with a little cayenne

Cold boiled salmon mixed with low-cholesterol margarine and seasoned with a little sea salt

Shrimps on lettuce, with sliced hard-boiled egg

Mussels and cucumber

Marmite

Cold minced lamb with chopped onion or chives, or grated celery.

Anyone with heart disease, or overweight, is advised to avoid salted fish.

Hot toasted sandwiches

Chicken club sandwiches

Toast slices of wholemeal bread. Spread with low-cholesterol margarine and place a thin slice of roast chicken on one piece. Season with sea salt, then cover with a lettuce leaf dipped in yoghurt. Cover with another slice of toast and press together. Cut in triangles and serve hot.

Crab toast

Mash the crab meat and season with sea salt and chopped chives. Spread one slice of toast with this mixture, then press the other slice on top. Cut in triangles and serve with the claws of the crab as decoration. Lobster meat may be treated in the same way.

Fisherman's luck sandwiches

Toast slices of wholemeal bread and spread with low-cholesterol margarine. Cook the fish (mackerel, halibut, or some other white fish), lay a thin slice on a piece of toast and sprinkle with grated horseradish. Lay a second slice of fish on top and sprinkle this with cider vinegar. Place the second slice of toast on this, and press lightly together.

Sweet sandwiches

To satisfy a sweet tooth, choose from the following:

Any diabetic jams, except those containing citrus fruits.
Honey
Mashed banana
Date and ginger: chop finely and combine the following ingredients; ½ cup stoned dates, ½ cup walnuts, and ¼ cup preserved ginger.

8

Salads

Due to forced immobility, a large percentage of arthritic patients are overweight. This causes increased pain because of the extra pressure put on those painful joints, especially in the lower parts of the body – the lower spine, hips, knees, ankles and feet. In my opinion, eating less and counting calories is not the answer. Our meals must provide materials for the three main purposes, namely, growth and repair of body tissues, energy and warmth, and protection and maintenance of good health. The following salads are easy to prepare and contain all three properties.

Margaret Hills' special

1 red pepper, cored and seeded
1 green pepper, cored and
   seeded
100 g (4 oz) cashew nuts
1 large red eating apple
½ small cauliflower, washed
   and dried
4 large spring onions, washed
   and dried
1 cup cold cooked wholegrain
   rice
home-made French dressing
   (see page 51)

Chop red and green peppers, apple, onions and cauliflower into very small pieces, add cashew nuts and cooked rice. Toss in home-made French dressing.

Cold meat salad

slices of cold lamb or poultry
1 hard-boiled egg, chopped
a few capers
lettuce leaves, or watercress
chopped parsley
4 cooked potatoes, cut small
sea salt and pepper
home-made mayonnaise (see
   page 51)

Arrange a border of lettuce or watercress on a plate. Cut the meat into neat pieces and add to them the egg, capers, parsley, and potatoes. Season. Add to the centre of the plate and pour on home-made mayonnaise.

Chicken salad

cold cooked chicken
lettuce leaves
½ cucumber
watercress
cooked green peas

beetroot
hard-boiled egg
home-made mayonnaise (see
    page 51)

Cut the chicken meat into neat pieces. Wash and thoroughly dry the lettuce and arrange in a salad bowl with slices of cucumber, a few peas, slices of beetroot, and the chicken. Just before serving, pour on some home-made mayonnaise and garnish with quarters of hard-boiled egg and watercress.

Cottage cheese salad

100 g (4 oz) cottage cheese
    (per person)
lettuce

peach slices
a few grapes
a few radishes

Thoroughly wash and dry the lettuce and arrange the leaves on a plate. Top with several peach slices, grapes and radishes. Serve the cottage cheese in a separate dish. Complete the meal with a slice of wholemeal bread spread with low-cholesterol margarine, a crisp eating apple and a glass of skimmed milk.

Sardine salad

tin of sardines
1 hard-boiled egg
½ teaspoon made mustard
watercress
6 cold cooked potatoes

1 beetroot
2 tablespoons sunflower oil
1 tablespoon cider vinegar
sea salt

Make dressing by mixing oil, vinegar, mustard and salt. Arrange sliced potatoes and beetroot in a salad bowl and pour on the dressing. Place the drained and boned sardines on the top. Garnish with watercress and sliced egg.

Fish salad

cold cooked white fish
lettuce
hard-boiled egg
a few capers
a few gherkins

a few shrimps
aspic jelly
home-made mayonnaise (see
    page 51)

Flake the cooked fish, taking great care to remove all bones. Separate the yolk from the white of the hard-boiled egg, and chop the white only. Put the fish into a bowl and add shrimps, chopped white of egg, a few capers, shreds of gherkins. Mix together and pour on the home-made mayonnaise. Wash and dry lettuce leaves and arrange in a border on a plate. Place the fish salad in the centre, garnish with watercress, chopped aspic and yolk of egg passed through a sieve.

Russian salad

350 g (12 oz) or more of cold,
    cooked vegetables,
    including green peas,
    young carrots, French
    beans, turnips, potatoes,
    cauliflower
6 olives
1 tablespoon capers
2 gherkins
300 ml (½ pint) home-made
    mayonnaise (see page 51)

2 anchovies
1 tablespoon minced parsley
1 hard-boiled egg
1 teaspoon tarragon and
    chervil, mixed
sea salt
pinch of soft brown sugar

Cook the vegetables in the usual way in salted water, then cut the carrots and turnip into dice. Slice up the French beans finely. Dice the potatoes and break the cauliflower into tiny florets. Put the vegetables into a bowl and add hard-boiled egg chopped up finely. Pound the anchovies and add them. Mix well together and season with herbs, parsley, sea salt, and sugar. Pour in the mayonnaise and blend together. Transfer to a salad dish and decorate with capers, gherkins and olives.

Lettuce salad

1 lettuce	mustard
½ beetroot, cooked	1 tablespoon cider vinegar
¼ Spanish onion	1 tablespoon corn oil
cress	½ teaspoon light muscovado
1 hard-boiled egg	sugar
sea salt	

Chop the yolk of the hard-boiled egg and add salt, a little mustard and the cider vinegar. Mix together and then add the corn oil, sugar and chopped white of egg. Shred the lettuce leaves into a salad bowl. Add sliced onion, cress and sliced beetroot, and then pour on the dressing. Serve to accompany cold meat, with slices of wholemeal bread spread with low-cholesterol margarine.

Summer salad

lettuce	young radishes
mustard and cress	cucumber

Cut lettuce, radishes and cucumber into thin slices. Arrange in a salad bowl and garnish with mustard and cress. Sliced hard-boiled egg may be used as additional garnish and flaked cold fish mixed into the salad makes this a tasty lunch.

Winter salad

endive	beetroot, cooked
mustard and cress	celery
1 hard-boiled egg	salad dressing

Shred the celery into thin pieces and arrange with endive and cress in centre of bowl. Garnish with sliced beetroot and sliced hard-boiled egg. Add salad dressing to taste. Serve with cold meat or poultry and baked jacket potato.

SALAD DRESSING

Mayonnaise dressing

3 tablespoons sunflower oil	1 yolk of egg
1 tablespoon cider vinegar	pinch of sea salt

Separate the yolk from the white of the egg. Put the yolk into a bowl with the salt. Stir it with a wooden spoon. Add the oil very gradually, a drop at a time, stirring it into the egg. A little more may be added slowly, although never more than a few drops at a time. The mixture should become smooth and thick. Finally the cider vinegar should be added in the same way, drop by drop, and stirring constantly. The dressing should be quite smooth.

French dressing

3 tablespoons sunflower oil	sea salt
1 tablespoon cider vinegar	1 teaspoon each of mint,
1 teaspoon clear honey	parsley, chives, thyme – all
1 teaspoon finely chopped onion	chopped finely

Combine all the ingredients in a screw-topped jar, adding sea salt to taste, and shake well to blend.

Yoghurt dressing

100 g (4 oz) natural yoghurt	1 teaspoon clear honey
1 tablespoon cider vinegar	sea salt

Place ingredients in a bowl, add sea salt to taste and mix thoroughly.

9

Meatless Dishes

There is nothing to beat fresh vegetables for supplying the body with the vitamins, minerals and trace elements needed to return it to a state of health and maintain a healthy condition. Vegetables should be eaten raw as far as possible; otherwise they should either be steamed or boiled in a little water containing a small pinch of sea salt, and the water used to make gravy or drunk as a cocktail. This way none of the valuable water-soluble vitamins are lost.

Cold vegetable savoury

Although left-over vegetables can be used for this salad, it is nicer if you cook them specially and mix them with hot cooked rice, then allow the mixture to cool. This is excellent with fish.

4 hard-boiled eggs	50 g (2 oz) peas, cooked
6 spring onions, or ½ onion, chopped	100 g (4 oz) unpolished rice, cooked
1 red pepper, chopped	150 ml (¼ pint) oil and cider vinegar dressing

Coarsely chop the hard-boiled eggs. Mix chopped onions, pepper and peas into rice. Pour on oil and cider vinegar dressing and mix well. Finally mix in chopped eggs. Serve cold.

Wholewheat pancakes

100 g (4 oz) wholemeal flour	150 ml (¼ pint) skimmed milk and/or water
a good pinch of sea salt	
1 egg	

Sieve the flour and salt into a basin. Make a well in the centre and drop in the egg. Add about half the liquid, a little at a time, and mix from the middle outwards. Beat well until the mixture is smooth and creamy. Add the rest of the liquid and beat again. Heat a little corn oil in a frying pan and pour in a small amount of batter. Tilt the pan until it is evenly covered, and cook quickly until the pancake is golden brown underneath. Then toss, and brown the other side.

Pancakes can be stuffed with sautéed vegetables for a savoury dish, or covered in apple sauce or similar filling for a sweet.

Omelette

Per person

2 eggs, beaten	1 teaspoon water
a pinch of sea salt and pepper	25 g (1 oz) low-cholesterol margarine

Add water to the beaten eggs and season with salt and pepper. Melt the margarine in an omelette pan. When the margarine 'sizzles' pour in the eggs. Do not shake the pan, but pass a fork around the side to loosen the eggs, then gently work them back, lifting the sides, and turning the centre, so that the liquid eggs on top can run to the bottom of the pan. Tip the pan up from the handle, urge the omelette slightly forward and the omelette will shape. Tip on to a hot plate and serve.

Variations:

Potato and onion omelette

Fry diced potato and chopped onion in melted low-cholesterol margarine until cooked. Add to omelette when cooked before folding over.

Spanish omelette

Add cooked vegetables, chopped up, to the egg mixture before making omelette, e.g. onion, red pepper, green pepper, potato, carrot, courgette, etc.

Mushroom omelette

Add cooked mushrooms to cooked omelette before folding over.

Chicken omelette

Warm leftover chicken thoroughly in a white sauce and add to cooked omelette before folding over.

Quick paella

2 tablespoons corn oil
50 g (2 oz) low-cholesterol
  margarine
1 onion, chopped
4 mushrooms, chopped
sea salt and pepper

1 red or green pepper, diced
100 g (4 oz) peeled prawns
175 g (6 oz) long-grain
  unpolished rice, cooked

Put the oil and margarine in a large frying pan. Fry the onion and mushrooms and add the remaining ingredients. Toss well and heat through for about 5 minutes.

Mushroom pancakes

25 g (1 oz) low-cholesterol
  margarine
450 g (1 lb) mashed potatoes
sea salt and pepper

1 onion, finely chopped
50 g (2 oz) mushrooms, finely
  chopped

Heat the margarine in a frying pan. Add the potato, season well, smooth, add onion and mushrooms and cook gently until crispy brown underneath – about 10 minutes. Fold over with a palette knife and slide on to a plate.

Mushroom casserole

225 g (8 oz) mushrooms,
  quartered
1 tablespoon dried parsley
1 small onion, diced
900 ml (1½ pints) vegetable stock

6 tablespoons corn oil
1 bay leaf
450 g (1 lb) barley

Sauté mushrooms, parsley, onion and barley in oil. Put into a casserole dish with bay leaf and a pinch of sea salt and pepper. Add stock and bake at 180°C/350°F/Gas Mark 4 for about 45 minutes, until barley is tender and liquid absorbed.

Cabbage and celery casserole

2 oz corn oil
1 small onion, peeled and
sliced
1 small head celery, washed
and sliced

½ small white cabbage,
shredded

For the sauce

25 g (1 oz) wholemeal flour
25 g (1 oz) low-cholesterol
margarine
300 ml (½ pint) skimmed milk

sea salt and pepper
25 g (1 oz) fresh wholemeal
breadcrumbs

Heat the oil in a frying pan. Add the onion and celery and cook gently for 5 minutes, stirring from time to time. Add the cabbage and allow to simmer on a gentle heat for a further 5 minutes. Melt the margarine in a saucepan and add the flour to make a roux. Add the skimmed milk gradually, stirring with a wooden spoon until a smooth sauce is formed. Season well. Turn the vegetables into a 1.2 l (2-pint) casserole dish and season well. Pour on the sauce and sprinkle with breadcrumbs. Dot the surface with margarine and cook in the oven at 180°C/350°F/Gas Mark 4 for 20 minutes, until the crumb topping is golden brown.

Mixed vegetable casserole

50 g (2 oz) low-cholesterol
margarine
2 large onions, thinly sliced
4 new carrots, thinly sliced
1 turnip, thinly sliced
1 leek, sliced
2 potatoes, thinly sliced

225-g (8-oz) packet frozen corn
and peppers
sea salt
freshly ground black pepper
300 ml (½ pint) stock

Melt the margarine in an ovenproof casserole. Toss in the sliced onions and leave on a low heat for about 5 minutes. Add the other vegetables with seasoning between each layer. Pour in the stock. Cover the casserole and cook in the oven for 45 minutes, at 180°C/350°F/Gas Mark 4, or until the vegetables have absorbed the stock.

Potato and lentil hotpot

225 g (8 oz) lentils
750 g (1½ lbs) potatoes
3 onions, sliced
2 oz corn oil

1 dessertspoon yeast extract
450 ml (¾ pint) warm water
sea salt and pepper

Put layers of onions, lentils and sliced potatoes into a pie dish, seasoning between the layers and nearly filling the dish. Finish with potatoes. Dissolve the yeast extract in water and pour over. Dot with oil and cover. Bake in a moderate oven for about one hour, at 180°C/350°F/Gas Mark 4, or until tender, then brown without a lid. Serve with green vegetables.

Cottage cheese fritters

100 g (4 oz) plain wholemeal
  flour
½ teaspoon sea salt
1 egg, separated

5 tablespoons water
225 g (8 oz) cottage cheese
corn oil, for frying

Sift flour and salt into a bowl, make well in centre and break egg yolk into it. Work flour into egg yolk, gradually adding water at the same time. Beat thoroughly. Beat in the cottage cheese. Whisk egg white until just stiff and fold lightly into cottage cheese mixture. Heat oil in a frying pan. Drop in four separate tablespoons batter and cook over moderate heat until golden brown underneath. Turn over and cook on other side. Remove and drain on kitchen paper. Keep hot. Repeat, to make approximately 16 fritters. Serve with a little honey.

Cottage cheese flan

20-cm (8-inch) cooked
  pastry flan case,
  made with 100 g (4 oz)
  wholemeal flour,
  50 g (2 oz) low-cholesterol

margarine, ½ teaspoon sea
salt, and 2 tablespoons
water

For filling

1 large onion	150 ml (¼ pint) skimmed
15 g (½ oz) low-cholesterol	milk
margarine	225 g (8 oz) cottage cheese
1 tablespoon capers	8 anchovy fillets
2 eggs, beaten	sea salt and pepper

Warm the pastry flan case through in the oven. Chop onion finely and fry until golden brown in margarine. Add the chopped capers, beaten eggs, milk and cottage cheese. Season. Turn into the hot flan case and decorate with a lattice of anchovy fillets. Bake in a moderate oven, at 180°C/350°F/Gas Mark 4, for 20 minutes on centre shelf until set.

Potato and onion pie

900 g (2 lbs) potatoes	sea salt and pepper
225 g (8 oz) onions	50 g (2 oz) low-cholesterol
	margarine

Peel the potatoes thinly and slice 5-mm (¼-inch) thick. Peel and slice the onions. Cover with cold, salted water and bring to boil. Simmer gently for about 5–7 minutes, or until cooked. Drain well and dry. Layer the potatoes and onions in a greased shallow pie dish. Season each layer. Dot with margarine and brown under grill.

10

Meat Dishes

The leanest cuts of meat should always be chosen and any extra fat trimmed off before cooking. The skin should be removed from chicken and turkey. Expensive cuts are not necessary – lean minced lamb is excellent. Always use sunflower oil for browning meat and vegetables for a casserole, and skim off any fat that appears.

A wok is an extremely useful addition to the kitchen since it can be used for steaming – by placing the food on a plate on a trivet or using stacked bamboo steamers. Chinese cuisine is a very healthy diet in that careful attention is given to the correct balance of ingredients. Very little meat is used and vegetables predominate. Stir-frying can be done in a minimum of corn oil and all the flavour and goodness are retained. I have included here a few Chinese dishes – so easy to cook and absolutely delicious.

Roast lamb

Joints to choose: best end of neck, breast (this is an economical but rather fat joint to be boned, covered with a stuffing, then rolled), leg, loin, saddle (this is a double loin and ideal for parties), or shoulder.

Allow 20 minutes per 450g (1lb) weight and 20 minutes over at 220°C/425°F/Gas Mark 7 for the first 30–45 minutes, then lower the heat to 190–200°C/375–400°F/Gas Mark 5–6 for the rest of the time.

Serve lamb with mint sauce: mix finely chopped mint leaves with cider vinegar and muscovado sugar to taste.

Rolled shoulder of lamb

1 shoulder of lamb, boned
1 teaspoon sea salt
½ teaspoon pepper
6 tablespoons wholemeal
  breadcrumbs

40 g (1½ oz) low-cholesterol
  margarine
1 tablespoon chopped parsley
1 egg

Mix in a bowl the pepper, salt, breadcrumbs and margarine. Add to this the chopped parsley, and bind all together with the egg. Place this stuffing into the shoulder where the bone has been removed, and roll the meat into a neat roll, tying it loosely around, as the bread in the stuffing will swell during cooking. Roast in hot oven, 220°C/425°F/Gas Mark 7, and allow 15 minutes per 450 g (1 lb) and 15 minutes over. Serve with brown gravy.

Grilled lamb chops

6 lamb chops

oil or melted low-cholesterol
  margarine

Preheat grill. Brush the meat with oil or melted margarine. Season well and place under grill. Cook under hot grill for about 10 minutes turning occasionally during grilling. Serve with green salad.

Lamb hot pot

2 tablespoons corn oil
2 tablespoons wholemeal flour
sea salt and pepper
450 g (1 lb) onions, peeled and
  sliced
2–3 carrots, peeled and sliced
2 sticks celery, sliced
1 leek, sliced
300 ml (½ pint) stock

900 g (2 lbs) middle neck of lamb,
  cut into 2.5-cm (1-inch) cubes
1 teaspoon Worcestershire sauce
1 teaspoon rosemary, finely
  chopped
15 g (½ oz) low-cholesterol
  margarine
450 g (1 lb) potatoes, peeled and
  sliced
parsley, finely chopped

Heat the oil in a frying pan. Coat lamb in seasoned flour and brown in the oil. Add the onions and celery and reduce the heat for 5 minutes. Layer the lamb in a casserole with the onion mixture, carrots and leek, finishing with the potatoes. Pour in stock, Worcestershire sauce and rosemary. Season well. Dot with margarine, cover and cook for 2 hours at 180°C/350°F/Gas Mark 4. Remove the lid for final 45 minutes of cooking time. Garnish with chopped parsley.

Shredded lamb with noodles and spring onions

100 g (4 oz) transparent noodles
1 egg
1 tablespoon cornflour
1½ tablespoons water
225 g (8 oz) lean lamb, shredded
3 tablespoons corn oil

2 tablespoons soy sauce
4–5 spring onions, cut into pieces
300 ml (½ pint) chicken stock
1 tablespoon sesame seed oil

Soak the noodles in hot water for 5 minutes; drain. Beat the egg with the cornflour and water. Add the lamb and turn to coat. Heat the oil in a pan over high heat. Add the lamb and stir-fry for 1 minute. Sprinkle in the soy sauce and spring onions and stir-fry for 1 minute. Add the stock and noodles and bring to the boil, stirring. Simmer for 5 minutes. Sprinkle with the sesame seed oil and simmer for 1 minute. Serve hot.

Fried lamb slices with onions

225 g (8 oz) lean boned lamb, thinly sliced
½ teaspoon sea salt
1 teaspoon cornflour
4 tablespoons corn oil

225 g (8 oz) onions, sliced
2 garlic cloves, crushed
2 tablespoons soy sauce
1 teaspoon sesame seed oil

Mix the lamb slices with the salt and cornflour. Heat the corn oil in a wok or frying pan. When it is very hot, add the lamb and stir-fry until lightly browned. Remove from the pan with a slotted spoon and set aside. Add the onions and garlic to the pan and fry until just tender. Return the lamb to the pan with the soy sauce. Stir well. Add the sesame seed oil just before serving. Serve hot.

Roast veal

Veal is an exceptionally lean meat and must be kept well basted with corn oil during cooking. It also needs adequate cooking. Joints to choose: best end of neck, breast, fillet, chump end of loin or loin shoulder.

Allow 25 minutes per 450 g (1 lb) weight and 25 minutes over at 220°C/425°F/Gas Mark 7 for the first 30–45 minutes, then lower the heat to moderate, 190°C/375°F/Gas Mark 5 for the rest of the time.

Serve veal with bread sauce (made with 1 small onion soaked in warm skimmed milk for approximately 15 minutes, add ½ cupful of wholemeal breadcrumbs, stir and season to taste), and thickened gravy.

Veal chops

8 thin loin chops
sea salt and pepper
25 g (1 oz) low-cholesterol
   margarine

1 teaspoon parsley, finely
   chopped
1 dessertspoon cider vinegar

Wipe chops and sprinkle with sea salt and pepper. Grill under preheated grill, turned low, for 8–10 minutes each side. Blend margarine with parsley and cider vinegar. Put the margarine to cool after reshaping into a rectangle. Place chops on a hot plate and garnish with blended margarine. Serve immediately.

Blanquette de veau

900 g (2 lbs) breast of veal
sea salt and pepper
a little grated nutmeg
1.2 l (2 pints) veal stock, or
   water and skimmed
   milk
bouquet garni

1 onion
1 clove
a little wholemeal flour
50 g (2 oz) low-cholesterol
   margarine
4–5 mushrooms
bay leaf

Cut up the veal into neat pieces and put into a saucepan with stock or water and milk to cover. Add the onion stuck with clove, also the bouquet garni and bay leaf. Season to taste. Bring to boiling point, skim well, then simmer for 1 hour. Strain off the liquid and keep. Dissolve the margarine in a saucepan, stir in the flour, cook but do not brown. Moisten this with a little veal stock. Add this to the whole liquid, reheat, season with salt, pepper and nutmeg, if desired. Add the pieces of veal and heat through. Add the mushrooms. Serve in pyramid form with a border of peas.

Liver à la Française

450 g (1 lb) lamb's liver, sliced
3 tablespoons wholemeal
  breadcrumbs
4 mushrooms, chopped
1 onion, finely chopped
2 sprigs of parsley, finely
  chopped

½ teaspoon sea salt
pinch each of pepper and
  nutmeg
300 ml (½ pint) stock
Worcestershire sauce

Grease a casserole dish well. Mix together breadcrumbs, mushrooms, onion, parsley, salt, pepper and nutmeg. Sprinkle this over each piece of liver and place in casserole dish. Add stock and bake in oven, 160°C/300°F/Gas Mark 2, for ¾ hour. Arrange liver and vegetables on hot dish. Add a little Worcestershire sauce to gravy, boil up and pour round liver. Toasted wholemeal breadcrumbs may be sprinkled on top as garnish.

Stewed lamb's liver

225 g (½ lb) lamb's liver
25 g (1 oz) low-cholesterol
  margarine
25 g (1 oz) wholemeal flour
300 ml (½ pint) stock or water

2 onions
1 apple
1 potato
sea salt and pepper

Melt the margarine in a saucepan. Cut the liver into small pieces and coat in seasoned flour. Fry the liver a rich brown, then remove the liver and brown the remainder of the flour, adding the stock gradually and stirring till it boils. Return the liver to the sauce and add the vegetables, peeled and diced. Simmer gently for 1 hour, season and serve very hot.

11

Poultry and Game

The meat of poultry and game is an excellent source of protein and should be eaten freely. The skin, however, is full of cholesterol and should be removed and discarded.

Guinea fowl with tartare sauce

guinea fowl
low-cholesterol margarine,
   melted

tartare sauce (see below)
sea salt
watercress

Clean and prepare the bird, and split it in half. Brush it over with melted margarine and season well. Place the halves in a grill pan and cook gently under a preheated grill until golden brown, turning as necessary. Serve on a bed of watercress with tartare sauce.

Tartare sauce

1 teacup mayonnaise, home-
   made with cider vinegar
   (see page 51)

1 tablespoon chopped gherkins
   or capers
½ teaspoon finely chopped
   shallot (optional)

Mix the gherkins, or capers, and shallot, if used. Add to the home-made mayonnaise. Add a little seasoning, if necessary.

Devilled chicken legs

3 tablespoons corn oil
1 tablespoon Worcestershire
  sauce
1 tablespoon cider vinegar
1 tablespoon finely chopped
  onion

1 teaspoon French mustard
sea salt
4 chicken legs
100–225 g (4–8 oz) mushrooms
1 tablespoon corn oil
parsley

Mix all the ingredients for the sauce together: corn oil, Worcestershire sauce, cider vinegar, onion, mustard. Season. Score the chicken legs with a sharp knife and place in a grill pan. Brush with the sauce and place under a hot grill. Grill for 8–10 minutes, basting frequently with the sauce. Turn, brush with more sauce and continue grilling for a further 8–10 minutes, or until cooked. Brush the mushrooms with oil and add to the grill pan for the last 5 minutes cooking time. Serve hot, garnished with parsley, and accompanied by a salad.

Chicken pilau

2 onions
1 clove garlic (optional)
2 tablespoons oil
225 g (8 oz) long-grain
  whole rice
600 ml (1 pint) chicken stock,
  made by simmering chicken
  carcass or giblets

25–50 g (1–2 oz) sultanas
few pine nuts or other
  (optional)
350 g (12 oz) diced
  cooked chicken meat
sea salt
crisp breadcrumbs, for
  garnish

Peel and chop the onions, crush the garlic. Fry in the hot oil for a few minutes, then add the rice, turning in the oil. Add the stock, bring to the boil and stir. Simmer, uncovered, for about 10 minutes. Add the rest of the ingredients, then cook for a further 10–15 minutes until the liquid has just been absorbed. Pile on to a hot dish and top with a garnish of crisp breadcrumbs or nuts. Serve with salad or a green vegetable.

Farmhouse chicken

1.5-kg (3-lb) chicken
40 g (1½ oz) low-cholesterol
   margarine
2 sticks celery, sliced
2 carrots, sliced

300 ml (½ pint) stock
sea salt
6 small onions, sliced
1 small turnip, sliced

Melt the margarine in a pan and fry the chicken lightly on all sides. Transfer to a casserole dish, add the sliced vegetables, stock and seasoning. Cover and cook for about 1½ hours until tender, at 190°C/375°F/Gas Mark 5, basting occasionally with the stock. Thicken gravy if necessary before serving.

Roast duck and apple sauce

1 duck, oven ready
sage-and-onion stuffing

apple sauce (see below)
watercress

Wipe the duck and insert the sage-and-onion stuffing. Roast on a rack in the oven, 15 minutes per 450 g (1 lb) and 15 minutes over at 220°C/425°F/Gas Mark 7, reducing to 180°C/350°F/Gas Mark 4 after half an hour. Baste well during cooking. Serve the duck on a hot plate, with a watercress garnish and apple sauce.

Apple sauce

450 g (1 lb) cooking apples
   water

25 g (1 oz) low-cholesterol
   margarine
honey

Peel, core and slice the apples. Put into a saucepan with a little water and cook to a pulp. Beat smooth and add the margarine and a little honey to taste.

Raised game pie

750 g (1½ lbs) wholemeal flour
175 g (6 oz) low-cholesterol
   margarine
300 ml (½ pint) water
1 egg

900 g (2 lbs) game, i.e. pigeon,
   pheasant, or rabbit
a little sea salt

Cut the game meat into small pieces, season with sea salt. Boil the water and margarine together. Pour into the centre of the flour. Mix to a stiff dough, knead well, then set aside to cool a little. Mould into shape, put the game in the centre, cover with pastry. Decorate the lid, brush over with beaten egg, make a hole in the centre and bake in oven at 180°C/350°F/Gas Mark 4 for approximately 1½ hours.

Chicken with peppers

225 g (8 oz) chicken breast meat, boned and skinned
1 tablespoon cornflour
2 slices ginger root, peeled
2 spring onions
4 tablespoons corn oil
½ teaspoon sea salt

1 egg white
1 green pepper, cored and seeded
1 red pepper, cored and seeded
2 chillis, seeded
2 tablespoons black bean sauce

Cut the chicken meat into cubes. Mix the cubes with, firstly, the sea salt, then the egg white and finally the cornflour. Cut the green and red peppers into small square pieces. Slice ginger root, spring onions and chillis. Heat the oil in a wok or frying pan and stir fry the chicken over a moderate heat, separating the cubes. Cook until lightly coloured, then remove with a perforated spoon. Increase heat under wok and when the oil is really hot put in the ginger root, chillis and spring onions, then add green and red peppers. Continue to stir for approximately 1 minute, then add the black bean sauce and return the chicken cubes to the mixture. Stir well for approximately 2 minutes and serve at once on a hot dish.

12

Sweets and Desserts

I always feel that a meal is not complete without a pudding or dessert to follow, and in my opinion nothing can equal a fresh fruit salad; a variety of fresh fruit of your choice and within the limits of your diet, washed carefully, cubed, and served in a fruit dish with a little low-fat ice cream, or custard made with skimmed or dried milk.

Baked apples

large eating apples
chopped nuts and raisins

low-cholesterol margarine
honey

Core the apples, wash well and fill the cavity with chopped nuts and raisins. Put a small piece of low-cholesterol margarine on top of each and place in a baking dish. Bake for about 1 hour at 180°C/350°F/Gas Mark 4, add honey to taste, if required, and serve hot. Custard made from skimmed or dried milk is a delicious extra.

Baked whole rice

2/3 cups unpolished whole rice
1.2 l (2 pints) skimmed milk

1 tablespoon honey
½ teacup raisins

Mix rice, milk and honey and stir in the washed raisins. A little low-cholesterol margarine may be added if desired. Bake in oven at 200°C/400°F/Gas Mark 6 for about 1 hour, stirring the pudding occasionally during the first half hour.

Baked bananas

Take 3 bananas (weight about 450g/1 lb), bake them for 20 minutes at 200°C/400°F/Gas Mark 6, and serve hot with custard or low-fat ice cream.

Banana trifle

4 sponge cakes
300 ml (½ pint) skimmed
  milk
300 ml (½ pint) custard,
  made with skimmed
  or dried milk

2 bananas
50g (2 oz) dates
almond flavouring

Add a little flavouring to milk and heat in a pan. When hot pour over sponge cakes. Slice the bananas and arrange on top and then pour over hot custard. Decorate with dates, cut into quarters.

Coconut pudding

2 slices stale wholemeal bread
2 heaped tablespoons
  desiccated coconut
600 ml (1 pint) skimmed milk

1 or 2 eggs, separated
25g (1 oz) low-cholesterol
  margarine
50g (2 oz) melted honey
  sugar

Cut up the bread into small square pieces. Grease a pie dish with plenty of margarine and fill with alternate layers of bread and coconut. Beat the yolks of the eggs slightly and add to them the milk and honey. Pour this over the dry ingredients and bake in a moderate oven, 180°C/350°F/Gas Mark 4, for 30 minutes, or until set. In the meantime, whip the whites of eggs stiffly, and stir in a little sugar. Pile this roughly over the pudding, sprinkle with coconut and return to the oven to set.

Treacle pudding

225 g (8 oz) wholemeal flour
75 g (3 oz) low-cholesterol
    margarine
150 ml (¼ pint) skimmed milk

3 tablespoons molasses
1 dessertspoon ground
    ginger
½ teaspoon carbonate of soda

Put flour into a basin, add margarine and chop finely into flour with a knife. Dissolve the soda in some of the milk and add with the molasses and the rest of the milk. Mix thoroughly, put into a greased basin and simmer for two hours. Serve with a sweet pudding sauce (see page 73).

Fruit Tart

any fruit (apples, peaches,
    pears, bananas, apricots)
honey

water
shortcrust pastry (see page 79)

Prepare the fruit, half fill the pie dish. Add honey to taste and a little water and top up with rest of the fruit. Roll out the pastry and cut out the top of the pie. Brush the edges of the dish with water and line them with strips of pastry, moisten the strips and then place pastry on the top of the pie. Press the edges together and trim. Work the edges up with a knife and decorate them. Brush over the tart with water, or whipped white of egg, sift with demerara sugar and bake at 200°C/400°F/Gas Mark 6, for about half an hour. Serve hot or cold.

Summer pudding

any suitable fruit, i.e. apples,
    peaches and pears
honey

thin slices of stale bread
custard sauce (see page 73)

Stew the fruit with honey to taste. Line a pudding basin with thin slices of bread, fitting to a round at the bottom. Pour in the stewed fruit gradually, allowing the bread to get well soaked with the syrup. Place on top a round of bread, cover with a plate and allow to stand till quite cold and set. Turn out and serve with thick custard sauce.

Apples à la crème

6 apples
3 whites of eggs
2 tablespoons honey

300 ml (½ pint) water
cherries and angelica
low-fat ice cream

Put the apples in a dish with the honey and water and bake gently until soft, at 180°C/350°F/Gas Mark 4. When cold cover with stiffly beaten white of eggs and bake till set. Decorate with cherries and angelica. Serve with ice cream.

Almond pudding

75 g (3 oz) ground almonds
600 ml (1 pint) skimmed milk
2 eggs

50 g (2 oz) honey
65 g (2½ oz) ground rice
50 g (2 oz) browned almonds

Mix the ground rice with a little milk. Boil the remainder of the milk, pour over the rice, return to the pan and stir till it thickens. Add 40 g (1½ oz) ground almonds, beaten eggs, honey and some of the browned almonds. Oil a pie dish, line it with the remainder of ground almonds, pour in the mixture, bake for 15 minutes, 180°C/350°F/Gas Mark 4, sprinkling the top with a few browned almonds.

Cinnamon pudding

450 g (1 lb) apricots
50 g (2 oz) honey
2 teaspoonfuls cinnamon

225 g (8 oz) wholemeal
  breadcrumbs
2 eggs

Soak the apricots and then stew till quite soft. Rub through a sieve. Mix all the ingredients together, pour into an oiled pudding basin or mould. Steam for 45 minutes and serve with a sweet pudding sauce (see page 73).

Milk jelly

600 ml (1 pint) skimmed milk   25 g (1 oz) honey
25 g (1 oz) gelatine   any flavouring

Soak the gelatine in a little of the milk for 20 minutes. Add the honey to the rest of the milk and bring to the boil, stirring. Allow to cool slightly, then stir in the dissolved gelatine. Mix well. Flavour or colour to taste. Rinse out a jelly mould in cold water then pour in the liquid. Put in a cool place to set. (This makes a very good dish for an invalid.)

Custard sauce

300 ml (½ pint) skimmed milk   15 g (½ oz) cornflour
1 egg   15 g (½ oz) honey

Mix the cornflour with a little of the milk, put the rest on to boil. When boiling, stir in the cornflour and cook for 3 minutes, then add the honey. Allow to cool a little, then add the beaten egg. Stir till it thickens, but do not allow to boil again. Add flavouring if required.

Sweet pudding sauce

25 g (1 oz) low-cholesterol   15 g (½ oz) honey
    margarine   vanilla or almond essence
15 g (½ oz) wholemeal flour
300 ml (½ pint) skimmed milk

Melt the margarine, add the flour and cook it for 1 minute. Stir in the milk and simmer gently for 5 minutes. Then add honey and flavouring.

Chocolate sauce

½ level tablespoon cornflour   vanilla essence
½ level tablespoon cocoa   15–25 g (½–1 oz) low-cholesterol
300 ml (½ pint) skimmed milk   margarine
1 tablespoon demerara sugar

Blend the cornflour and cocoa with a little cold milk. Heat the remainder of the milk and when boiling pour on to the blended mixture. Return to the heat and cook for 2–3 minutes, stirring continuously. Add the sugar, a few drops of vanilla essence and the margarine. Serve hot.

13

Cakes and Biscuits

It is very likely that the fat used in shop-bought cakes, pastry and biscuits is of the saturated type which must be avoided. This does not mean that you cannot have these treats – you can still enjoy delicious home baking using low-cholesterol margarine, muscovado sugar or honey for sweetening, and skimmed or dried milk. If you are watching your weight it is best to avoid these foods except on rare occasions. Although it is advisable to limit your egg intake, remember you will be eating only a very small proportion of egg yolk in a small slice of cake.

Mrs Lyne's sunflower cake

225 g (8 oz) wholemeal
  self-raising flour
175 ml (6 oz) sunflower oil

175 g (6 oz) raw cane sugar
2 eggs
100 g (4 oz) sultanas

Mix oil and sugar together, beat in eggs, add flour and fruit. Cook for 1 hour 10 minutes at 170°C/320°F/Gas Mark 3.

Nut and raisin loaf

225 g (8 oz) wholemeal
  self-raising flour
½ teaspoon sea salt
a pinch of bicarbonate of soda
25 g (1 oz) muscovado sugar

50 g (2 oz) chopped nuts
75 g (3 oz) raisins
1 dessertspoon clear honey
6 tablespoons skimmed milk
  (approx.)

Sieve the flour, salt and bicarbonate of soda into a bowl, add the sugar, chopped nuts and raisins and mix together. Gradually beat in the honey, and milk and mix well to a wet dough. Place the mixture in a well-greased loaf tin (about 7.5 × 18 cm/3 × 7 inches) and bake at 180°C/350°F/Gas Mark 4 for about 40 minutes. Slice thinly and serve with butter.

Date loaf

275 g (10 oz) wholemeal flour
50 g (2 oz) chopped walnuts
225 g (8 oz) dates, chopped
175 g (6 oz) muscovado sugar
1 tablespoon low-cholesterol
   margarine
a pinch of sea salt
1 egg
vanilla essence
boiling water

Mix dates, sugar and margarine. Pour on 300 ml (½ pint) boiling water. Beat up the egg and add to the mixture, together with flour and walnuts. Season with one teaspoon vanilla essence and a pinch of sea salt. Mix and pour into a well-greased baking tin and bake at 180°C/350°F/Gas Mark 4 for about 45 minutes.

Wholemeal gingerbread

350 g (12 oz) wholemeal flour
100 g (4 oz) muscovado sugar
40 g (1½ oz) mixed peel
100 g (4 oz) low-cholesterol
   margarine
1 teacup black molasses
½ teacup skimmed milk
½ teaspoon baking soda
2 teaspoons ground ginger
1 egg

Mix flour, mixed peel and ginger. Heat sugar, molasses and margarine in saucepan until dissolved. Mix well with flour, and add beaten egg. Warm the milk, dissolving the baking soda in it, and add to the mixture. Bake at 180°C/350°F/Gas Mark 4 for 1¼ hours.

Honey cheesecake

225 g (8 oz) wheatmeal biscuits
50 g (2 oz) low-cholesterol
   margarine
350 g (12 oz) cottage cheese
100 g (4 oz) honey
2 teaspoons Barbados sugar
2 eggs
a pinch of sea salt
ground cinnamon

Crush the biscuits and mix with the melted margarine. Press around the inside edge and over the bottom of a 20-cm (8-inch) sandwich tin. Chill. Beat the cheese, honey, sugar, eggs and salt together until smooth and spoon into the biscuit crumb shell, sprinkling liberally with cinnamon. Cook for 35–45 minutes in the centre of oven, 150–160°C/275–300°F/Gas Mark 1–2. Allow to cool in oven.

Sponge cake without fat

3 large eggs
100 g (4 oz) Barbados sugar
25 g (1 oz) melted
low-cholesterol margarine
(if the cake is to be kept
for a day or two)

75 g (3 oz) wholemeal self-
raising flour
1 tablespoon hot water

Put the eggs and sugar into a basin and whisk until thick. Sieve the flour and fold in gently and carefully with a metal spoon. Fold in water and the margarine, if used. Divide the mixture between two greased and floured 18-cm (7-inch) sandwich cake tins and bake near the top of a hot oven, 220°C/425°F/Gas Mark 7. Test by pressing gently in the centre; if firm the sponges are cooked. Remove from the oven and turn on to a wire tray to cool.

Arrowroot biscuits

50 g (2 oz) arrowroot
100 g (4 oz) wholemeal flour
1 egg

25 g (1 oz) Barbados sugar
75 g (3 oz) low-cholesterol
margarine
1 teaspoon baking powder

Rub the margarine into the flour, then add the sugar and arrowroot. Finally, add the baking powder and egg. Roll out the mixture and cut into shapes. Bake at 190°C/375°F/Gas Mark 5, until firm.

Kringles

50 g (2 oz) low cholesterol
margarine
4 egg yolks, 1 egg white

50 g (2 oz) Barbados sugar
225 g (8 oz) wholemeal flour

Melt margarine gradually over boiling water. Break 4 egg yolks into a basin with 1 egg white, and beat well. Add to eggs the sugar and margarine. Stir with wooden spoon till quite smooth. Add flour and mix to a stiff paste. Knead paste well on a floured board. Roll out to 1-cm (½-inch) thickness and cut into shapes. Prick with fork dipped in flour. Bake for 10–15 minutes at 190°C/375°F/Gas Mark 5. If liked brown, brush with egg first.

Danish honey rings

225 g (8 oz) wholemeal flour
a pinch of sea salt
150 g (5 oz) low-cholesterol
margarine
25 g (1 oz) ground almonds

1 egg, beaten
4 tablespoons clear honey
1 family block low-fat ice
cream

Sieve the flour and salt into a bowl, rub in margarine until mixture resembles fine breadcrumbs. Stir in ground almonds and mix together with egg and honey. Place dough in a large piping bag with a 'star' pipe. Pipe mixture into rings on greased baking sheets. Bake in the centre of oven at 220°C/425°F/Gas Mark 7 for 8–10 minutes. Remove and leave to get cold. Serve sandwiched with ice cream.

Coconut biscuits

225 g (8 oz) desiccated coconut
50 g (2 oz) Barbados sugar

75 g (3 oz) ground rice
whites of 3 eggs

Mix together the dry ingredients. Whip egg whites to stiff froth. Add a little at a time to mixture and mix well. Put in very rough heaps measured with a tablespoon on a well-greased baking sheet. Bake at 220°C/425°F/Gas Mark 7 for 5 minutes, then allow oven to cool to 160°C/300°F/Gas Mark 2, and cook slowly for 30 minutes approximately. The biscuits should be a golden brown.

Raisin scones

350 g (12 oz) wholemeal flour
25 g (1 oz) low-cholesterol
   margarine
sea salt

450 ml (¾ pint) skimmed milk
   (approx.)
175 g (6 oz) raisins
2 teaspoons baking powder

Rub margarine into sieved flour, baking powder and a little salt. Add raisins, then milk to make a soft dough. Roll out to about 2.5 cm (1 inch) thick and cut into rounds. Brush over with a little milk and bake at 230°C/450°F/Gas Mark 8, for 12–15 minutes.

Wholemeal shortcrust pastry

225 g (8 oz) wholemeal flour
100 g (4 oz) low-cholesterol
   margarine
1 tablespoon water

sea salt
yolk of 1 egg

Rub the margarine into the flour. Add the water and a pinch of salt. Mix with beaten egg yolk and add water if required. Roll out and use.

Flapjacks

100 g (4 oz) low-cholesterol
   margarine
25 g (1 oz) muscovado sugar

4 level tablespoons clear honey
225 g (8 oz) rolled oats

Melt the margarine with the sugar and honey in a large pan. Add the oats and mix well. Spread the mixture smoothly over a 20 × 30-cm (8 × 12-inch) tin and bake in the centre of oven at 180°C/350°F/Gas Mark 4, for 15–20 minutes, or until golden brown and firm to the touch. Mark into squares or fingers while warm, but allow to cool in the tin, then remove carefully.